The Inflammation Syndrome

*The Complete Nutritional Program
to Prevent and Reverse Heart Disease,
Arthritis, Diabetes, Allergies, and Asthma*

Jack Challem

WILEY

John Wiley & Sons, Inc.

Published by John Wiley & Sons, Inc., Hoboken, New Jersey
Published simultaneously in Canada

The Inflammation Syndrome™ and Anti-Inflammation Syndrome™ are trademarks of Jack Challem.

Table on page 42 is from S. B. Eaton and S. B. Eaton II, "Paleolithic vs. Modern Diets—Selected Pathophysical Implications," *European Journal of Nutrition* 39, no. 2 (2000): 67–70. Reprinted with permission.

Quick Chicken or Turkey Rice Soup recipe on page 94 was adapted with permission from Helen Smith and Melissa Diane Smith.

For general information about our other products and services, please contact our Customer Care Department within the United States at (800) 762-2974, outside the United States at (317) 572-3993 or fax (317) 572-4002.

Wiley also publishes its books in a variety of electronic formats. Some content that appears in print may not be available in electronic books. For additional information about Wiley products, visit our website at www.wiley.com.

Library of Congress Cataloging-in-Publication Data:
Challem, Jack.
    The inflammation syndrome : the complete nutritional program to prevent and reverse heart disease, arthritis, diabetes, allergies, and asthma / Jack Challem.
        p.   ;   cm.
Includes bibliographical references and index.
    ISBN 0-471-20271-1 (cloth)
    ISBN 0-471-47881-4 (paper)
    1. Inflammation—Diet therapy.   2. Inflammation—Alternative treatment.
3. Chronic diseases—Etiology.
    [DNLM: 1. Inflammation—diet therapy—Popular Works.   2. Anti-Inflammatory Agents—Popular Works.   3. Autoimmune Diseases—diet therapy—Popular Works. QW 700 C437i 2003]   I. Title.
    RB131 .C475   2003
    616'.0473—dc21   2002014015

Printed in the United States of America
10   9   8   7   6

In memory of Harold G. Miller,
teacher, mentor, and friend.

CONTENTS

FOREWORD

Occasional injuries are part of the human experience, and healing is the body's self-repair process. Healing begins with inflammation, which nature meant to clean up damaged tissues and protect against infection. So if inflammation is beneficial, why are so many modern diseases characterized by chronic and unhealthy inflammation?

The Inflammation Syndrome answers a big part of this important question. Chronic inflammation underscores and promotes virtually every disease, affecting millions of people, and yet inflammation also is a symptom rather than the fundamental cause of these diseases. When we dig deeper, we find that chronic inflammation is the consequence of an injury to the body combined with nutritional imbalances or deficiencies. To properly treat inflammatory diseases, it is essential to correct the underlying dietary problems.

We speak from experience. At the Center for the Improvement of Human Functioning International, physicians, nurses, and other staff members have focused on these objectives for more than twenty-seven years. We use careful clinical and laboratory workups—what is now termed evidence-based medicine—to assess the health, nutritional reserves, and biochemical uniqueness of each patient. We have successfully treated people from around the country and around the world, many of whom were considered untreatable or incurable by conventional medicine.

Through these detailed individual workups, we have gained an understanding of chronic, or sustained, inflammation. More often than not, individuals with chronic inflammation, such as with arthritis and asthma, have low levels of anti-inflammatory antioxidants (such as vitamins E and C), omega-3 fatty acids, and many other important nutrients. Many patients also have previously undetected adverse food reactions, abnormal gut permeability, yeast overgrowth, and hormonal imbalances. All of these factors can impair normal functioning of the immune system, sustaining inflammation well beyond its biological usefulness.

The pharmaceutical perspective of inflammation focuses on relieving symptoms through over-the-counter analgesics and far more powerful prescription drugs. Inflammation does not result from a deficiency of aspirin, cortisone, or Cox-2 inhibitors. Rather, as *The Inflammation Syndrome* so well documents, there is a desperate need to address the basic nutritional influences on chronic inflammation. After all, no drug can ever make up for a nutritional deficiency. Under these circumstances, it becomes paramount to feed a person's biochemistry with the best nutrition.

This is where measuring a patient's nutrient levels proves to be so helpful in confirming the underlying nutritional and biochemical causes of inflammation and motivating patients to action. It would be easy to lecture a patient on the anti-inflammatory effects of good nutrition, omega-3 fatty acids (which include fish oils), or vitamin E. But a far more powerful motivator is testing and demonstrating the patient's low levels.

By doing so, we have found time and again that such hard evidence is extremely persuasive. This meaningful individual information, combined with the ease of dietary improvements and supplementation, empowers patients with knowledge and motivates them toward self-healing. Patients develop the attitude, "I want my levels to be optimal," and then they work toward achieving them. Furthermore, from our medical perspective, laboratory testing enables us to later recheck nutrient values to confirm proper absorption and utilization.

Through testing, we have realized that no one can ever assume that a person's diet is adequate. For example, a cardiac surgeon would never simply hope his patient's potassium level is sufficient to prevent fatal arrhythmias during heart surgery; he ensures that it is. The same approach applies to the treatment of chronic inflammation. To achieve optimal levels of many nutrients, one must often consume levels of vitamins, minerals, and other nutrients above those "officially" recommended for health. There is nothing wrong in doing so, especially when tests have shown patients to be low in these nutrients. At the very least, erring on the side of modest excess provides a margin of safety, a dose of nutritional insurance.

Jack Challem, the author of *The Inflammation Syndrome,* is a gifted health writer with a profound understanding of the role good nutrition plays in health. He has written a sound and practical book of benefit to anyone with chronic inflammation. As we read and discussed his book, we visualized Jack working in a huge lighthouse. The light being emitted is the cumulative scientific evidence so deftly organized and clearly presented here. The danger is the jagged rocks of chronic, sustained inflammation, which underlie almost every serious health issue facing modern society—and the reason for the lighthouse. All of us—readers, patients, and physicians alike—are piloting our own boats and, as a society, we are heading for the rocks. Will we see the light? Can we avoid the forces making us drift in the dark? To survive, we must rediscover the great Hippocratic ideal: Let food be thy medicine.

—Ronald E. Hunninghake, M.D.
Medical Director
The Olive W. Garvey Center for Healing Arts
Wichita, Kansas

—Hugh D. Riordan, M.D.
President
The Center for the Improvement of
Human Functioning International, Inc.
Wichita, Kansas

ACKNOWLEDGMENTS

Many individuals made major and minor contributions to this book. I thank Melissa Diane Smith, who helped renew my interest in wholesome foods and coached me in the kitchen before I began this book. The chapters relating to diet and recipes would not have been possible without her influence.

My sincere appreciation and thanks go to my agent, the late Michael Cohn, and my editor at John Wiley & Sons, Tom Miller, for their commitment to this book's message. I also thank Kimberly Monroe-Hill and William Drennan for their careful copyediting of this book, especially Kimberly's editing of my recipes.

I thank Hugh D. Riordan, M.D., and Ronald E. Hunninghake, M.D., for their encouragement, advice, and kindness.

I thank Hunter Yost, M.D., Malcolm Riley, D.D.S., and Bill Thomson for their reading of the initial manuscript and their excellent suggestions for improvement.

I thank Mary Larsen for her careful reading of the finished manuscript.

I also thank Burt Berkson, M.D., Ph.D., Ashton Embry, Matt Embry, Victor A. Feddersen, Abram Hoffer, M.D., Ph.D., Richard P. Huemer, M.D., Judy Hutt, N.D., Robert Ivker, D.O., Richard Kunin, M.D., Shari Lieberman, Ph.D., Soren Mavrogenis, and the others who kindly contributed case histories.

Special thanks go to Claus Gehringer, Ph.D., Björn Falck Madsen, and Eddie Vos for sharing ideas and pointing out research that I would otherwise have missed.

Introduction

One condition explains your stiff fingers, aching muscles, and arthritic joints. One condition lies at the root of your troublesome allergies and asthma. And one condition describes the underlying cause of heart disease, Alzheimer's disease, and some types of cancer.

It is *inflammation*.

As you read this, medicine is rapidly redefining coronary artery (heart) disease, the leading cause of death among people in the United States and most other Westernized nations, as an inflammatory disease of the blood vessels. Physicians are quickly adopting a new and inexpensive blood test—high-sensitivity C-reactive protein—to measure their patients' level of inflammation and risk of suffering a heart attack. And as the evidence mounts, physicians and medical researchers are recognizing that other major chronic diseases are fueled by inflammation as well.

Most of us understand inflammation as something that causes redness, tenderness, stiffness, and pain. It is the core of inflammatory "-itis" disease, and it also is intertwined in every disease, including obesity, diabetes, and multiple sclerosis.

Inflammation is why professional athletes and weekend warriors often development muscle aches. It is why some people's gums bleed whenever they brush their teeth. And it is why some people develop stomach ulcers.

Despite their different symptoms, all of these health problems are united by the same thread: they have runaway inflammation in common.

And as you may well realize, many people suffer from more than one inflammatory disorder. This constellation of related diseases, such as the combination of heart disease, arthritis, and periodontitis, can best be described as the Inflammation Syndrome.

—⊗—

Estimated Number of North Americans with Some Inflammatory Diseases

Millions of North Americans suffer from inflammatory disorders, some of which have only recently been recognized as inflammatory in nature:

Allergic and nonallergic rhinitis	39 million
Asthma	17 million
Cardiovascular diseases	60 million
Arthritis (all types combined)	70 million
Osteoarthritis	21 million
Rheumatoid arthritis	2 million

—⊗—

Everyone experiences inflammation at one time or another, and we actually need it to survive. But *chronic inflammation* is a sign that something has gone seriously awry with your health. Instead of protecting and healing, chronic inflammation breaks down your body and makes you older and more frail.

Most people treat inflammation with one or more over-the-counter or prescription drugs. At best these drugs temporarily mask the symptoms of inflammation, not treat its underlying causes. Worse, the side effects of these drugs can often be extraordinarily dangerous, causing weight gain, severe stomach pain, bone deformities, and heart failure.

Unfortunately, a physician's diagnosis of many -itis diseases, such as dermatitis or gastritis, is often meaningless. The doctor might feel proud of his diagnosis, but it is merely a description of the symptoms, not of its cause.

To understand the cause of the modern epidemic of inflammatory diseases, we have to look at how the average person's diet has deteriorated over the past two or three generations. The bottom line is that the foods you eat have a powerful bearing on your health and, specifically, inflammation.

How does food influence your inflammation, your aches and pains?

Your body is a remarkable biological machine, designed to make an assortment of pro- and anti-inflammatory substances. What you eat—proteins, carbohydrates, fats, vitamins and vitaminlike nutrients, and minerals—provides the nutritional building blocks of these substances. Some nutrients help form your body's inflammation-promoting compounds, which normally help fight infections. Others help produce your body's anti-inflammatory substances, which moderate and turn off inflammation.

Until recently, people ate a relative balance of pro- and anti-inflammatory nutrients. Today, because of extensive food processing, our diet has become seriously unbalanced. The typical Western diet now contains at least thirty times more of pro-inflammatory nutrients than just a century ago. As a result, people have become nutritionally and biochemically primed for powerful, out-of-control inflammatory reactions. An injury, infection, or sometimes nothing more than age-related wear and tear create the spark that, in a manner of speaking, sets your body on fire.

The Inflammation Syndrome reveals many of the hidden dangers in foods that set the stage for inflammation, worsen aches and pains, and increase the long-term risk of debilitating and life-threatening diseases. This book explains how and why inflammation eats away at your health. For example:

- Common cooking oils, such as corn, safflower, and soy oils, can make arthritis and asthma worse.
- Fries and other deep-fried foods, breakfast bars, and cookies can interfere with your body's innate ability to control inflammation.
- Corn-fed beef, promoted as healthy, is far worse than grass-fed beef and can aggravate your inflammation.
- Not eating your vegetables or taking your vitamins can increase breathing problems in people with asthma.
- Being overweight increases your body's production of inflammation-causing substances.
- Taking common anti-inflammatory drugs will actually make your osteoarthritis far worse.
- If you have one inflammatory disease, you are likely to develop others in the coming years, because the inflammation will eventually spread and affect other parts of your body.

I have had my own experience with inflammation and how I have avoided chronic pain. Several years ago, while in the British Museum in London, I paid careful attention to a sign reading "Mind the Step." Unfortunately for me, the area was not well lit and the sign failed to warn me of a second step. I tripped and seriously injured my right foot. The pain was so excruciating that I almost passed out. I sat down while my head cleared and, I had hoped, for the pain to ease.

It didn't. By the next morning, my entire foot was literally turning black and blue. Although no bones were broken, I did give myself one of the most serious types of muscle strain. A couple of days later, on the next leg of my trip, in France, I hobbled around at a scientific conference on antioxidant vitamins. Climbing into the shower was an ordeal, as was putting on my socks and shoes. My foot had swelled, its color was awful, and I was taking aspirin several times daily to reduce the inflammation, swelling, and pain.

Weeks later, at home, my foot had regained its normal color and, by all outward signs, had healed. However, I still felt a sharp pain in the foot whenever I walked. I realized that this injury, if it did not heal soon and properly, could lead to a lifetime of chronic inflammation and pain. Frustratingly, all of the vitamin supplements I had been taking for years didn't seem to help. And then it dawned on me. That scientific meeting in France was about a well-known herbal antioxidant made from French maritime pine bark (called Pycnogenol), and the scientific literature showed it to have powerful anti-inflammatory effects. I started taking it, and within days the pain went away. To rule out the power of suggestion, I stopped taking the supplement for a few days, and the pain returned. I started taking the supplement again and the inflammation and pain went away and have never returned. I walk and hike long distances without any discomfort in the foot.

The Inflammation Syndrome does not simply dwell on the problem of inflammation. Most of this book coaches you on how to avoid the foods that make you more susceptible to information and to instead select foods that can reduce inflammation and your risk of many diseases. *The Inflammation Syndrome* describes a new way of viewing inflammatory disorders as a consequence of eating an unbalanced diet.

You will learn plenty of practical information about how to prevent and reverse inflammation. The book's Anti-Inflammation Syndrome Diet Plan describes

- the dietary imbalances that lead to chronic inflammation;
- a balanced, nutritious diet plan to reduce inflammation;
- tasty recipes and guidelines for making your own anti-inflammatory meals;

- the best natural anti-inflammation supplements, such as fish oils, vitamin E, herbs, and many others;
- case histories of patients treated by nutritionally oriented practitioners.

You may wonder why you should trust the advice of someone who is not a physician.

The reason is simple, though it may surprise you: while I believe the majority of physicians are sincere and well-meaning, most do not understand the fundamental role of nutrition in health. Medical schools teach virtually nothing about the practical, preventive, and therapeutic uses of nutrition and supplements. The doctors I write about in this book are notable exceptions to this rule in that they are both sincere *and* have an understanding of nutrition.

For more than twenty-five years, I have been reading scientific and medical journals; talking with nutritionally oriented biologists, biochemists, and physicians; and writing about how vitamins, minerals, and other aspects of nutrition can greatly improve health. I have also published original research articles in medical journals, something rare for nutrition writers. Though I am not a medical scientist, I have a solid understanding of the science behind the health benefits of nutrition and supplements.

In many ways, *The Inflammation Syndrome* expands on the concepts described in my previous book *Syndrome X: The Complete Nutritional Program to Prevent and Reverse Insulin Resistance*. Far more than genes, poor eating habits are at the core of most modern degenerative disorders, including chronic inflammation. *The Inflammation Syndrome* is supported by hundreds of scientific studies and by successful clinical experiences, many of which you will read. Some of my scientific references are at the back of this book, and I encourage you to share all of them with your physician.

Ultimately, you alone are responsible for your own health. You cannot ignore your personal responsibility and simply turn your body over to a doctor the way you might ask a mechanic to fix your car. This book provides a plan for you to empower yourself to safely prevent and overcome inflammatory disorders. You will discover how easy it is to take charge of your diet and your health—and to feel better than you ever imagined.

PART I

The Inflammation-Disease Connection

CHAPTER 1

Meet the Inflammation Syndrome

Hank and Debra: The Deadly Effects of the Inflammation Syndrome

For Hank and Debra, what they didn't know came back to hurt them.

In college they were athletic, trim, and attractive. Hank was the star of the college football team, and Debra was an avid tennis player. Youth was on their side, and they quickly recovered from the inevitable athletic injuries.

After they graduated and married Hank pursued a career in sales, enjoying its competitive nature but not immediately recognizing how it kept him from exercising. Meanwhile, Debra juggled motherhood and periodic jobs to earn extra money. Like many people, they learned to save time by eating mostly ready-to-heat convenience foods and fast-food restaurant meals, which tended to be high in fat and carbohydrates and low in vegetables.

Hank regularly suffered from heartburn and indigestion, but he never figured out that his poor food choices were the source of his stomach upsets. Debra had developed asthma and mild rheumatoid arthritis. Both were prescribed medications by their physicians, but diet was never even considered a potential factor in their deteriorating health.

By middle age their trim athletic figures were little more than a memory. Hank had gone from a lean 180 to 250 pounds, and Debra's weight had ballooned from 110 to 180 pounds. Hank's blood cholesterol was elevated and, combined with his weight, significantly increased his risk for heart disease. He had also developed chronic aches and pains in his shoulders and hips, a result of old football injuries. Meanwhile, Debra's asthma and arthritis had gotten worse, and she was taking prednisone and other medications to control her symptoms.

In their fifties Hank developed adult-onset (type 2) diabetes and Debra was diagnosed with breast cancer. Hank was prescribed a glucose-lowering drug, and Debra underwent surgery and chemotherapy.

Having gone through all that, their health seemed relatively stable for several years. But retirement saw no relief for their health problems. Hank was taking eight prescription medications and Debra was taking six. At age sixty-two Debra's breast cancer reappeared, and treatment failed. She died at age sixty-three. Hank, who was largely confined to home (and had hot meals and groceries delivered by a local social service organization) had a heart attack and died at sixty-five.

All of Hank and Debra's health problems were treated according to the prevailing medical standards of care. But their doctors failed to see that poor food choices and chronic inflammation were intertwined in many of their health problems. As a result the doctors treated only symptoms, not the causes of Hank and Debra's problems.

Every disease, every ache, and every pain you suffer revolves around inflammation.

Inflammation is what causes the pain of arthritis, the discomfort of allergies, the wheezing of asthma, and the stiffness from overusing your muscles. Inflammation also underlies the most devastating and catastrophic of all diseases: heart disease, Alzheimer's disease, and many forms of cancer.

If that seems hard to believe, consider that over-the-counter anti-inflammatory drugs reduce the risk of heart attacks and Alzheimer's disease. But this book is not going to recommend that you take drugs to reduce inflammation. Their side effects all too often outweigh their benefits, especially when natural and safe anti-inflammatory foods and nutrients abound.

Even if you seem to be pretty healthy today, odds are that inflammation is simmering in your body, quietly damaging your heart, your mind, your organs. Such inflammation may be stirred up by physical injuries, frequent colds and flus, allergies, eating the wrong types of fats and car-bohydrates, and by having a "spare tire" around your middle. At a certain point your inflammation will boil over into painful and debilitating symptoms.

Inflammation is a normal process that can go dreadfully wrong. It is supposed to protect us from infections and promote healing when we are injured.

Chronic inflammation does just the opposite: it breaks down our bodies and makes us more susceptible to disease. Inflammation forces millions of people with arthritis to alter their daily lives, and it adds caution to the millions of people with asthma who do not know when their next suffocating attack will occur. Millions of other people—with multiple sclerosis, lupus, diabetes, and other disorders—also suffer from chronic inflammation.

The Inflammation Syndrome

Individual inflammatory disorders such as asthma or rheumatoid arthritis are bad enough. Far more insidious is the Inflammation Syndrome, the significance of which is only now being recognized in medical circles.

A syndrome is a group of symptoms that characterizes a particular disorder. For example, in my previous book *Syndrome X: The Complete Nutritional Program to Prevent and Reverse Insulin Resistance,* Syndrome X was defined as the clustering of abdominal fat, insulin resistance, hypertension, and elevated cholesterol—all of which significantly increase the risk of diabetes and coronary artery disease.

Similarly, the Inflammation Syndrome reflects the coexistence of at least two inflammatory disorders that significantly increase the risk of more serious inflammatory diseases. What causes this ongoing buildup in inflammation? Although an inflammatory response may primarily affect specific tissues, such as the knees, it commonly radiates through the body and randomly attacks other tissues. Over a number of years this systemic (bodywide) inflammation can contribute to diseases that might appear unrelated but that do share a common thread of chronic inflammation.

Some examples of the inflammation syndrome are in order. Let's start with being overweight, a condition that affects two-thirds of Americans and growing numbers of people in most other developed countries.

Excess weight contributes to inflammation because fat cells secrete chemicals, such as C-reactive protein and interleukin-6, that promote inflammation. Being overweight increases the risk of many other diseases, and part of the reason is related to inflammation. If you are overweight, you have a greater risk of developing adult-onset diabetes, which also has a strong inflammatory component. Inflammation in diabetes is related to being overweight, to having elevated blood sugar and insulin levels, and to consuming too many refined carbohydrates (such as white bread and sugary breakfast cereals).

The Inflammation Syndrome does not stop here. Having diabetes also increases the risk of periodontitis, a type of dental inflammation. Each of these disorders—overweight, diabetes, and periodontitis—is serious by itself. But as the inflammation in these disorders simmers year after year, it also increases the risk of coronary artery disease, which medicine has recently recognized as an inflammatory disease of the blood vessels. In a nutshell each inflammatory disorder has an additive effect, increasing the body's overall level of inflammation and the risk of very serious diseases.

Many other examples of the Inflammation Syndrome abound. Allergies stir up the inflammatory response, increasing the risk of rheumatoid arthritis, an autoimmune (self-allergic) disease. Infections also trigger an immune response, and chronic infections and inflammation account for an estimated 30 percent of cancers. Joint injuries frequently set an inflammatory response into motion, setting the stage for osteoarthritis. Serious head injuries and their resultant brain inflammation increase the long-term risk of Alzheimer's disease, which is also being viewed by doctors as an inflammatory process affecting brain cells.

This is serious and scary stuff, and the stakes for your health are very high. But the point of this book is that chronic inflammation and the inflammation syndrome can be prevented and reversed. This book shows you how.

What Is Chronic Inflammation?

Inflammation assumes many different forms, and everyone experiences it at one time or another. Perhaps the most common type of inflammation is sudden and acute, such as when you burn yourself in the kitchen, overuse muscles when moving furniture, or injure tendons when playing sports. The injured area swells, turns red, and becomes tender to touch.

Under normal circumstances inflammation helps you heal, and it can even save your life. For example, if you accidentally cut your finger with a knife, bacteria from the knife, air, or surface of your skin immediately penetrate the breach. Unchecked, these bacteria would quickly spread through your bloodstream and kill you.

However, your body's immune system almost immediately recognizes these bacteria as foreign and unleashes a coordinated attack to contain and stop the infection. Inflammation encourages tiny blood vessels in your finger to dilate, allowing a variety of white blood cells to leak out, track, and engulf bacteria. Some of these white blood cells also pick up and destroy cells damaged by the cut. In addition, inflammation signals the body to grow new cells to seal the cut. Within a day or two your cut finger becomes less inflamed, and a few days later it is completely healed.

Your body responds in similar fashion if you strain a muscle, such as by lifting too heavy a box, or by overexerting yourself during sports. The resulting inflammation, characterized by swelling, pain, and stiffness, is designed to remove damaged muscle cells and help initiate the healing process to replace those cells. Again, within a few days the inflammation decreases and you are well on the road to recovery.

Chronic inflammation, however, is very different. It does not go away, at least not quickly, and many people believe from their own experience that it will never go away. It results in persistent swelling, stiffness, or pain. Furthermore, you become more susceptible to inflammation as you age, but that, too, may be reversible.

—⚂—

QUIZ 1

How Is Your Current Health?

Have you been diagnosed with one of the following conditions, regardless of whether you are taking medications for treatment:

AIDS or HIV infection	*Add 2 points*	_____
Asthma	*Add 2 points*	_____
Bronchitis	*Add 1 point*	_____
Celiac disease or gluten intolerance	*Add 2 points*	_____
Coronary artery (heart) disease	*Add 2 points*	_____
Diabetes or elevated blood sugar	*Add 2 points*	_____
Gingivitis or periodontitis	*Add 1 point*	_____
Hepatitis	*Add 2 points*	_____
Inflammatory bowel disease	*Add 2 points*	_____

Rheumatoid arthritis　　　　　　　　　*Add 2 points* _____
Osteoarthritis　　　　　　　　　　　　*Add 2 points* _____
Eczema, psoriasis, or frequent sunburn　*Add 1 point* _____
Stomach ulcers　　　　　　　　　　　*Add 1 point* _____
Ulcerated varicose veins　　　　　　　*Add 2 points* _____
A recent physical injury—by accident, or through
　　sports/athletics, or via a severe sunburn　*Add 1 point* _____

Do you have any consistently stiff or aching joints, such as those in your fingers or knees?

Add 1 point _____

Does your body feel stiff when you get out of bed in the morning?

Add 1 point _____

If you are overweight by ten pounds or less, do you carry all or most of the extra fat around your abdomen?

Add 1 point _____

If you are obese (more than twenty pounds over your ideal weight), do you carry all or most of the extra fat around your abdomen?

Add 2 points _____

Is your nose stuffed up or runny a lot of the time?

Add 1 point _____

Do you get injured (anything from serious bruises to broken bones several or more times a year) because of accidents, the nature of your work, or athletic activities?

Add 1 point _____

Have you been hospitalized for surgery during the past twelve months?

Add 1 point _____

Do you smoke or chew tobacco products?

Add 2 points _____

Do you get frequent colds or flus?

Add 1 point _____

Do you have any seasonal allergies, such as to pollens or molds?

Add 1 point _____

Do you have any skin sores or rashes that don't seem to go away?

Add 1 point _____

Your score on quiz 1: _____

Interpretation and ranking:

0–1 **Low.** You have a low level of inflammation, which is healthy.

2–6 **Moderate.** You have a moderate level of inflammation that affects your current health and poses risks to your long-term health, and you should work to reverse it.

7–20 **High.** You have a high level of inflammation, which is very harmful and requires immediate attention to reverse.

21+ **Very high.** Although rare, your level of inflammation is extremely high and should be reversed without delay.

—ɱ—

Can Your Doctor Measure Inflammation?

For many disorders inflammation is so obvious it does not have to be measured. For example, the pain of arthritis is a clear enough sign of inflammation. Swelling, redness, and tenderness to the touch also are obvious signs of inflammation in muscle injuries, gingivitis, and many other disorders. These are typically localized forms of inflammation, though they burden the entire body with a variety of inflammation-promoting substances. Tests to confirm inflammation in these situations may be an unnecessary expense.

More general systemic, or bodywide, inflammation is not always apparent. Inflammation of blood vessel walls increases the risk of a heart attack, and inflammation of the stomach wall (gastritis) greatly increases the risk of ulcers and gastric cancer.

A common blood test measures the sedimentation rate (or "sed rate"), reflecting how fast red blood cells settle and form a sediment. Inflammation makes blood cells settle faster. The drawback to the sedimentation rate is that it is an extremely general indicator of inflammation.

Another test, called the high-sensitivity C-reactive protein (hs CRP) test, is a better indicator of systemic inflammation, though it still has the drawback of being a general indicator rather than pointing to a specific type of inflammation. Elevated CRP levels are associated with a 4.5 greater risk of having a heart attack, making it a far more accurate predictor than elevated cholesterol. Elevated CRP levels also are found in people with Alzheimer's disease, cancer, arthritis, acute infection, and physical trauma.

Recognizing Inflammatory Disorders

Physicians often speak in their own language, but it is actually very easy to identify most inflammatory diseases when you hear them in conversation or read about them. Most inflammatory diseases end with the suffix "-itis." For example, gastritis means inflammation of the stomach, tendinitis refers to inflammation of the tendons, and gingivitis means inflammation of the gingiva (gums).

At one time a physician's diagnosis typically included both the symptoms and the apparent cause of a disease. Unfortunately, that has changed, and the diagnosis of an -itis disease (and most other diseases as well) is now often nothing more than a description of symptoms. Dermatitis, an inflammation of the skin, can have many causes, including allergies, infections, a toxic reaction to a chemical, or abrasion. As good as you or your doctor might feel after a diagnosis, it is not likely that he or she will actually identify the underlying cause.

In the case of coronary artery disease something inflames blood vessel walls, triggering a cascade of events. That "something" might be a corrosive protein by-product called homocysteine, a low-grade infection, or oxidized cholesterol, all of which increase the risk of heart disease. (This relationship between inflammatory and cardiovascular disease will be discussed in depth in chapters 9 and 12.) In response, white blood cells migrate to artery walls, where they release free radicals, fuel inflammation, and exacerbate the damage. The most accurate predictor of whether you will have a heart attack is not your cholesterol, triglyceride, or blood sugar level. Rather, it is a high blood level of C-reactive protein, an indicator of your body's overall inflammation.

Common Inflammatory Diseases and Disorders

Inflammation is a symptom of virtually every disease process, and it often makes the condition worse. These are some examples of common disorders that involve inflammation:

Arthritis
  Osteoarthritis
  Rheumatoid arthritis
Injuries
  Athletic: tendinitis, bursitis, muscle strains, and bruises
  Cuts, broken bones, bruises, surgery

Infections
   Colds, flus, otitis media, hepatitis C, HIV, parasites, vague low-grade infections
Allergies/autoimmune
   Pollen and other inhalant allergies (rhinitis, nonallergic rhinitis)
   Food allergies
   Celiac disease (gluten intolerance)
   Lupus erythematosus
Pulmonary
   Asthma
   Chronic obstructive pulmonary disease
   Bronchitis
Cardiovascular
   Coronary artery disease, myocarditis, hypertension
   Phlebitis, varicose veins
Cancer
   Various types, including gastric, lung, breast, and prostate
Neurological
   Alzheimer's disease
Skin
   Sunburn (erythema)
   Eczema and dermatitis
   Psoriasis
Dental
   Gingivitis
   Periodontitis
Eye
   Conjunctivitis
   Uveitis
Digestive tract
   Gastritis, ulcers
   Crohn's disease
   Ulcerative colitis
   Diverticulitis
Miscellaneous
   Sinusitis
   Multiple sclerosis
   Obesity
   Diabetes

The Prevalence of Inflammation

One way to look at the prevalence of inflammatory diseases is to track sales (and, by implication, the use) of anti-inflammatory drugs such as aspirin, ibuprofen, naproxen sodium, and Cox-2 inhibitors. Each year more than 30 billion tablets of nonsteroidal anti-inflammatory drugs (NSAIDs) are sold over the counter in the United States—more than one hundred for every man, woman, and child. In addition, doctors write 70 million prescriptions for even stronger NSAIDs. Although some NSAIDs are often used to treat headaches (which may be caused by inflammation), these numbers reflect an enormous dependency on anti-inflammatory drugs.

Indeed, one of the pieces of evidence that coronary artery disease and Alzheimer's disease are inflammatory diseases is the fact that both may be prevented with some anti-inflammatory drugs. Aspirin reduces the risk of a heart attack, and ibuprofen (the active ingredient in Advil) appears to reduce the risk of Alzheimer's disease. Unfortunately, serious and sometimes life-threatening side effects are common from both drugs, which makes them undesirable approaches to prevention or treatment.

None of these drugs treats the underlying causes of inflammation. At best, they provide short-term relief. Worse, some NSAIDs hasten the breakdown of joint cartilage, increasing the damage and the progression of osteoarthritis. You will learn more about the dangers of anti-inflammatory drugs in chapter 5.

CHAPTER 2

Your Inflammation Triggers

Georgia: Allergies and Sinusitis

Georgia had suffered from chronic sinusitis, an inflammation or infection of the air spaces near the nose, since she was twelve, and developed asthma at age forty-one. She was also allergic to dust, grasses, smoke, perfumes, wool, and some cosmetics. Within a few years of her asthma diagnosis, Georgia was taking a variety of prescription drugs: oral and nasal, a bronchodilator, antibiotics, and other medications. She started to feel addicted to her asthma drugs and was afraid to be without them.

Her asthma was aggravated by the sinus problems, and Georgia found herself taking increasingly stronger medications. She also was having frequent and severe headaches. At age fifty-two, she consulted holistic physician Robert S. Ivker, D.O., of Denver, Colorado, author of several books, including *Sinus Survival, Asthma Survival,* and *Headache Survival.*

Ivker recommended a number of nutritional supplements, including vitamins E and C, beta-carotene, selenium, zinc, and an overall multivitamin, as well as a herbal echinacea and goldenseal combination. He also treated Georgia for candida infection and recommended that she purchase a negative-ion generator to improve the air quality in her home. These changes were combined with a tapering off of some of her medications and the beginning of a gradual exercise program, with walking and riding a stationary bicycle.

Two months after Georgia's first visit to Ivker, she had a new vitality and higher energy levels. She also had lost five pounds. Over the next year or so she was able to stop using all of her medications. Recognizing the role of emotion in illness, Ivker asked Georgia to focus on strengthening her family relationships. Today, with her newfound health, Georgia and her husband are planning for an active retirement.

Inflammation Triggers

Physicians and patients alike routinely confuse the *causes* of inflammation with its *triggers*. The causes of inflammation are often related to dietary imbalances or deficiencies, which prime the immune system for a powerful and chronic inflammatory reaction.

In contrast, inflammation triggers are the events that precipitate a specific inflammatory response *after* the body is already primed for an overreaction. Although it is not the same as correcting the causes of inflammation, it is very important to avoid events that trigger inflammation. Doing so helps settle down an easily agitated immune system.

First, try to reduce your exposure to inflammation triggers. For example, if you have food allergies, make a point of avoiding troublesome foods. Similarly, if you are a weekend-warrior athlete who frequently gets injured, it might be good to take up a more moderate and regular physical activity, such as swimming or walking. Repeated injuries keep revving up the body's inflammatory response.

Second, it is important to dampen the immune response to unavoidable triggers (e.g., seasonal pollen allergies). And third, it would be ideal to normalize the immune response to inflammation triggers. The second and third approaches rely chiefly on dietary changes and nutritional supplements, and these approaches are discussed in depth in later chapters.

For now, there are six general categories of inflammatory triggers to understand.

1. Age-Related Wear and Tear: What Is Your *Biological* Age?

Every living creature ages, and age is characterized by less biological efficiency and an accelerated breakdown of tissue and normal biochemical processes. When tissues break down white blood cells are mobilized to clean up, in a manner of speaking, the biological dust. The aging process occurs at individual rates of speed and is influenced by a variety of factors, including genetics, diet, frequency of infections, stress, and overall lifestyle. Of particular interest, levels of the body's key pro-inflammatory substances generally increase with age. This rise may be due to age-related tissue breakdown—and the immune system's response to it—or perhaps to the long-term effect of eating a pro-inflammatory diet.

Although most of us think of our age chronologically, our biological age is actually far more important. Chronological age refers to how many years old a person is, whereas biological age assesses age in terms of physical and mental performance. Many people in their seventies and eighties have more vigor and better health than do people half their age. Some researchers have noted that healthy centenarians are not simply healthy old people. They are often healthier than younger seniors and in many ways on a par with people in their forties.

One way to maintain a lower biological age is to reduce tissue break-down and the inflammation it stimulates. In a general way diets rich in vegetables and fruits provide large quantities of antioxidants, such as vita-min C, carotenoids, and flavonoids. These antioxidants neutralize damaging free radicals. For example, people who eat large amounts of antioxidant-rich vegetables develop fewer wrinkles and look younger. In a more specific example, many people take glucosamine sulfate supplements, which help maintain "younger" joints and reduce the pain of osteoarthritis.

2. Physical Injuries

Physical injuries can accelerate the aging of specific tissues, such as joints, muscles, and bone. Many such injuries, such as falling and break-ing a bone, or musculoskeletal athletic injuries, can become the source of painful and debilitating lifelong health problems. Former heavyweight boxing champion Muhammed Ali, who was physically and mentally agile as a young man, developed Parkinson's disease as a consequence of cumulative brain damage in the ring. These injuries become sources of chronic inflammation and pain because they are initially serious, re-peated, do not heal properly, or promote sustained low-grade inflamma-tion in the damaged tissues.

To minimize your chances of suffering a physical injury, you have to be careful of reckless behavior. For example, it's smart to drive defen-sively and to watch where you step, so you reduce the risk of tripping. As you reach middle age it may be better to adopt low-impact activities, such as swimming or walking.

3. Infections

In January 2002 researchers reported in the journal *Circulation* that repeated infections greatly increased a person's risk of dying from coronary artery disease. Literally, the more infections people experienced, the more likely they were to develop and die from heart disease. It wasn't that the bacteria and viruses were directly infecting the heart. More likely, repeated infections maintained a heightened activity of immune cells, which unleashed part of their damage on blood vessel walls.

Infections turn on the body's most powerful inflammatory responses, and sometimes the body ends up fighting itself. For example, a person who catches one cold after another suffers through a state of chronic inflammation with periodic peaks of inflammation, which slowly but surely attack and break down the entire body.

It is possible, nutritionally, to boost the *efficiency* of the immune system's response to infections. Vitamins C and E and a nutritional supplement called N-acetylcysteine (NAC) can greatly reduce the inflammatory symptoms of infections.

—∿—

Common Inflammation Triggers

Triggers prompt an inflammatory response when the body is already primed for such a reaction. These triggers do not cause an abnormal inflammatory reaction when the body is not primed for an overreaction.

Age-related wear and tear
  Lifelong breakdown of tissues
  Accelerated aging from poor dietary and lifestyle decisions
Physical injuries
  Repeated or severe athletic injuries
  Broken bones, cuts, wounds, burns, temporomandibular
  disease
Infections
  Frequent or chronic low-grade (e.g., colds and flus)
  Hepatitis or HIV
  Sepsis
  Chronic parasitic
Environmental stresses
  Sunburn, sunlight (ultraviolet rays)
  Tobacco, air pollution, lung irritants

Ionizing radiation
Cold air, exercise (asthma triggers)
Allergies and food sensitivities
   Pollen, mold, and other inhalant allergies
   Food sensitivities (may lead to ear infections), nightshades
   Cerebral allergies (affecting behavior and cognition)
   Celiac disease, gluten intolerance, lectin intolerance
Dietary imbalances and deficiencies
   Obesity (increases pro-inflammatory substances)
   Diabetes (elevates blood sugar)
   Inadequate vitamin C (increases blood vessel leakage)
   Inadequate B-complex vitamins (elevates homocysteine)
   Inadequate dietary antioxidants (stimulates inflammation)
   Imbalance in dietary fats (stimulates inflammation)

—m—

4. Environmental Stresses

Many common environmental stresses also can stimulate acute and chronic inflammatory responses. For example, tobacco smoke and other forms of air pollution irritate the lungs and activate large numbers of white blood cells, which contribute to further damage.

Cold air and exercise trigger severe asthma attacks in many people. The immune system of a person with asthma misreads the physiological changes triggered by cold air and exercise and overreacts to them. People with asthma are known to have abnormally high levels of free radicals, which prolong inflammation, but they can be reduced with such antioxidants as vitamin C and beta-carotene.

5. Allergies and Food Sensitivities

Pollen allergies, such as to ragweed, are common and have been increasing in prevalence. The most common allergenic pollens are from grasses, trees, and weeds, with sensitive people reacting when these plants release pollen into the air. Many people are also allergic to molds and dust. Their symptoms are collectively referred to as allergic rhinitis. About 15 percent of the North American population suffers from seasonal allergic rhinitis, and millions more people experience nonallergic rhinitis—basically nasal congestion or a runny nose unrelated to inhaled allergens.

Food sensitivities are allergiclike reactions. Some common allergies, such as to peanuts or shrimp, raise levels of IgE (immunoglobulin E), the conventional marker of an allergy. Beyond this, the topic of food allergies has often been charged with controversy because it has been difficult to identify a specific immune sign of a reaction. However, in recent years some physicians have found that many food allergies raise levels of IgG, which, like IgE, triggers a cascade of events that alter physical and mental health. Because blood tests may not always identify a specific immune reaction, you may have to rely on symptoms related to specific foods.

Nutritionally oriented physicians recommend strict avoidance of food allergens, and they often suggest that patients follow a "rotation diet" to reduce the likelihood of new food allergies developing. A rotation diet prohibits eating the same food or food from the same family (such as dairy) more often than once every four days. Sometimes allergic reactivity will diminish after several months of avoiding problematic foods.

Abnormal gut permeability may be created by an imbalance in various species of intestinal bacteria and the overgrowth of undesirable bacteria or yeasts such as *Candida albicans*. A "yeast infection," whatever the cause, can aggravate gut permeability, allergies, and inflammatory symptoms.

Maureen: Drugs Didn't Work

Maureen, a fifty-seven-year-old woman, had chronic but mild and manageable muscle and joint pains. She rarely ate tomatoes until her neighbor shared a bumper crop of tomatoes and eggplants, foods that are members of the nightshade plant family.

She soon began experiencing a significant increase in her joint pain, which was not relieved by anti-inflammatory medications. When Maureen related her health history to Hunter Yost, M.D., of Tucson, Arizona, he immediately recognized the likely cause of her increased pain: she is one of those people who is nightshade-sensitive.

Dr. Yost asked her to immediately stop eating all nightshades, which also include red and green peppers and potatoes. Within one week of eliminating all of these foods, Maureen had a significant decrease in joint pain, though her muscle pain did persist.

6. Dietary Imbalances and Deficiencies

Many dietary factors besides food allergies can lead to chronic inflammation. Being overweight—most often a consequence of either too many calories or too many carbohydrates—is a risk factor for many diseases, such as heart disease, cancer, diabetes, and osteoarthritis. The type of fat cells that develop around the abdomen generate large amounts of powerful inflammatory substances, such as C-reactive protein. Yes, obesity is an inflammatory disease.

An imbalance of dietary fats is a major promoter of inflammation. Many of the inflammation-sustaining fats are found in common cooking oils and packaged foods. When a balance of dietary fats is restored, through diet and supplements, the body regains its natural ability to both turn on and turn off inflammation.

Elevated blood sugar (glucose) levels, stemming from a diet with too many refined carbohydrates and sugars, also can increase inflammation in the body. People with insulin resistance commonly have high levels of C-reactive protein, a sign of inflammation. Insulin resistance is at the heart of Syndrome X and type 2 diabetes. Syndrome X, which increases the risk of both diabetes and heart disease, is also marked by fat around the waist, high blood pressure, and high cholesterol and triglycerides. For more information on Syndrome X see my earlier book *Syndrome X*.

The next chapter explains what happens during an inflammatory reaction, how the body makes powerful inflammation-producing substances from foods, and why many foods make us overreact to inflammation triggers.

CHAPTER 3

The Dietary Causes
of Inflammation

If injuries, infections, pollens, and other physical insults merely trigger inflammatory reactions, the obvious question is: What makes a normal process go out of control?

The answer lies in the foods we eat. If you eat the typical North American (or Western) diet, with abundant convenience and fast foods, you likely consume an unbalanced intake of the nutrients that promote inflammation. This imbalance results in large part from massive changes to our food supply over the past half century or so. During this time highly processed pro-inflammatory foods have largely replaced anti-inflammatory fresh and natural foods. The consequence has primed our bodies for chronic, excessive, and self-destructive levels of inflammation.

How do foods affect inflammation? The foods you eat provide the building blocks of your body and, of particular importance, your immune system, which regulates inflammation. Your immune system consists of dozens of specialized types of cells and molecules that constantly monitor your body for anything "foreign" or unusual. To envision this, it might help to picture how a taut, silken web alerts its resident spider to the presence of an insect. When a fly touches some threads in the web the resulting vibrations are transmitted and amplified throughout the web. These vibrations alert the spider, which moves in for the kill.

The cells of the immune system operate much like the interlocking filaments of the spider web. An immune cell senses the presence of an intruder (such as infectious bacteria or some other material, such as a damaged or dead cell) that does not belong in the body. An immune cell shares information about the peculiarity with other immune cells. Together they coordinate a response and, if the immune system is working properly, dispose of the foreign material.

You might wonder whether a powerful immune response is really necessary, but there is a biological rationale for it. Historically, infections have been the leading cause of human deaths. Even today, infections remain the third leading cause of death in the United States and the leading cause worldwide. A strong immune response gave us a fighting chance against infections. However, intense inflammatory responses are inappropriate when they target healthy tissues or harmless pollens, or when the body lacks normal switches to turn off inflammation.

Barbara: Inflammation, Rheumatoid Arthritis, and Asthma

At age forty-one, Barbara had suffered with rheumatoid arthritis and asthma for years and was taking half a dozen prescription drugs, which barely kept her symptoms in check. Then Barbara's physician started her on the hormone prednisone. After seven months on the drug she had gained 100 pounds—she was carrying 251 pounds on her 5'2" frame— and also developed the "moon face" characteristic of prednisone users. The cure was worse than the disease.

As a last-ditch effort, she went to a nutritionally oriented medical center in Wichita, Kansas. There, Hugh D. Riordan, M.D., and Ronald E. Hunninghake, M.D., found Barbara low in two essential "good" fats that are natural anti-inflammatory nutrients, as well as low in vitamins C and E and other nutrients. Lab tests also determined that Barbara had several allergylike food and chemical sensitivities, which helped fuel her overactive immune system and runaway inflammation.

The prescription was remarkably simple. Drs. Riordan and Hunninghake recommended that Barbara eat a more wholesome diet, avoid the foods and chemicals she was sensitive to, and take fish oil supplements (which contain the good fats) and vitamins. Nine months later, her asthma was completely gone, her arthritic symptoms were so mild that she reduced her prednisone to less than one-thousandth of the dose she had been taking—from 40 mg daily to 1 mg per month—and she was able to stop taking all the other medications. Barbara also had lost seventy pounds, and her outlook toward life changed as well. She was now energetic, upbeat, and outgoing.

Pro- and Anti-Inflammatory Counterbalances

With all the bad news we hear about fats, it may surprise you to read that some types of fats form the foundation of the body's pro- and anti-inflammatory compounds. Contrary to what you may have heard, fats (also known as fatty acids) are not inherently bad for health. Many fats are as essential for health as proteins, carbohydrates, vitamins, and minerals. Pro- and anti-inflammatory fats should serve as counterbalances to each other. Chronic inflammation can develop when there is a sharp imbalance in the types of fats consumed.

To understand how some fats increase or decrease inflammation, it helps to see them (and other pro- and anti-inflammatory substances) in simple terms, such as "matches" or "firefighters." Chronic inflammation often results from too many dietary matches. However, by making greater use of dietary firefighters you can restore a balance that prevents or even reverses chronic inflammation.

Pro-Inflammatory Matches

Two specific types of fats, as well as free radicals, prime our bodies for inflammation. Here is a brief description of them.

- The *omega-6* family of fatty acids supplies the building blocks of a variety of powerful pro-inflammatory substances. The omega-6 fatty acids are commonly found as *linoleic acid,* most often in vegetable oils such as corn, safflower, peanut, cottonseed, and soy oils, as well as in processed and packaged foods containing these oils. The omega-6 fatty acids stimulate the body's production of many other inflammation-causing chemicals, such as prosta-glandin E_2.
- *Trans fatty acids* are hidden in products containing "partially hydrogenated vegetable oils," including salad dressings, breakfast bars, shortening, nondairy creamers, stick margarines, and many baked items such as cakes and cookies. Omega-6 vegetable oils are bad enough in themselves, but hydrogenation gives them many of the characteristics of saturated fats. Trans fatty acids do much of their damage by interfering with the body's handling of anti-inflammatory fats, specifically the omega-3 fatty acids.
- *Free radicals* are hazardous molecules that damage the body's cells, increase the risk of many diseases, and accelerate the aging process. They also stimulate and prolong inflammatory reactions.

Anti-Inflammatory Firefighters

Three specific types of fats, as well as antioxidant nutrients, help control inflammation. Here is a brief overview of them.

- The *omega-3* family of fatty acids supplies the building blocks of a variety of powerful anti-inflammatory substances. The parent fat of the omega-3s, *alpha-linolenic acid,* is found in dark green leafy vegetables and flaxseed. More potent omega-3s, especially EPA (eicosapentaenoic acid), are found in coldwater fish such as salmon and herring. Basically, the omega-3s encourage the body's production of inflammation-suppressing compounds. They help remind the body to turn inflammatory reactions off when they are no longer needed.
- *GLA (gamma-linolenic acid)* is technically an omega-6 fatty acid, but it behaves more like an anti-inflammatory omega-3. It enhances the inflammation-suppressing effect of omega-3s.
- The *omega-9* family of fatty acids works with the omega-3s as anti-inflammatory compounds. They are found in olive oil, avocados, macadamia nuts, and macadamia nut oil.
- *Antioxidants* such as vitamins E and C are particular types of nutrients that neutralize free radicals and help quell inflammatory reactions.

The Pro-Inflammatory Pathway

Linoleic acid, the basis of all the other omega-6 fatty acids, is essential for health. However, the modern diet provides far too much of it, shifting our bodies toward chronic inflammation. The widespread use of vegetable cooking oils—in kitchens, restaurants, and packaged foods—is a principal reason for the prevalence of inflammatory disorders. As but one illustration, a study in the January 2002 *American Journal of Clinical Nutrition* showed that the omega-6 fats in vegetable oils increased inflammation in heart cells.

The body converts linoleic acid to a series of more powerful compounds. Chief among them is *arachidonic acid,* which is subsequently converted into a variety of very powerful inflammation-causing compounds known as *eicosanoids.* Eicosanoids include such substances as prostaglandin E_2.

The conversion of arachidonic acid to more powerful inflammation-causing substances such as prostaglandin E_2 is strongly influenced by a

—m—

Pro- and Anti-Inflammatory Pathways

OMEGA-6 FATTY ACIDS	OMEGA-3 FATTY ACIDS
Linoleic Acid	Alpha-Linolenic Acid
Found in margarine, shortening, and vegetable oils	Found in leafy vegetables, flaxseed, and fish
↓	↓
Production of pro-inflammatory compounds	Production of anti-inflammatory compounds

—m—

group of proteins called *cytokines*. Some of these cytokines, such as inter-leukin-6 (IL-6) and C-reactive protein (CRP), prompt cells to unleash a variety of pro-inflammatory compounds.

The Anti-Inflammatory Pathway

In parallel with linoleic acid, alpha-linolenic acid is the parent molecule of many of the body's anti-inflammatory firefighters. However, the omega-3 fatty acids are less active biologically, which places them at an immediate disadvantage against the omega-6 fatty acids. A person has to make an extra effort to consume foods or supplements rich in omega-3 fatty acids to compensate for their weaker activity.

The body uses various enzymes to convert alpha-linolenic acid to more active substances, particularly eicosapentaenoic acid (EPA). EPA is ultimately converted to a group of eicosanoids that are either anti-inflammatory or "less inflammatory" than those in the omega-6 family. The advantage of coldwater fish such as salmon or mackerel over other foods is that they contain large amounts of preformed EPA and docosa-hexaenoic acid (DHA), thus saving your body the time and effort needed to make them from alpha-linolenic acid.

If the diet is dominated by linoleic acid, as is the case with the typical modern Western diet, the body will make abnormally large amounts of inflammation-causing compounds. However, increased intake of alpha-linolenic acid or EPA will exert an anti-inflammatory effect.

Although GLA is technically a member of the omega-6 family, it behaves more like an anti-inflammatory omega-3 fatty acid. GLA increases the body's levels of the anti-inflammatory substance called prostaglandin E_1. It is among the body's checks and balances designed to prevent the omega-6s from getting completely out of control.

Considerable research has shown that people eating diets rich in alpha-linolenic acid, EPA, and DHA—think fish and vegetables—are less prone to inflammatory diseases. Research has similarly shown that supplements containing EPA, DHA, and GLA have striking anti-inflammatory properties in arthritis, allergies, asthma, and many other -itis diseases. This is why these fatty acids are the first-line supplements for preventing and reversing inflammation.

More Firefighters: Omega-9 Fatty Acids

Another group of fatty acids, known as the omega-9 family, also possesses impressive anti-inflammatory properties. Your body can make omega-9 fatty acids from other fats, assuming that things work the way they should, but some foods provide a direct source of them. The basic building block of the omega-9 fatty acids is oleic acid, a monounsaturated fat found abundantly in olive oil, macadamia nuts, and avocados.

Many studies have found that diets rich in olive oil reduce the risk or severity of inflammatory diseases such as coronary artery disease and rheumatoid arthritis. In general the omega-9 family is synergistic with the anti-inflammatory omega-3 family.

Skewing the Balance with Trans Fatty Acids

In human diets the ratio of omega-6 to omega-3 fatty acids has historically been in the range of 1:1 to 2:1. Today, omega-6 fatty acids dominate omega-3 fatty acids by ratios estimated between 20:1 and 30:1 in the typical Western diet. This lopsided intake of omega-6 fatty acids smothers the minuscule amounts of alpha-linolenic acid, EPA, and DHA found in most modern diets. The huge quantity of omega-6 fatty acids in the diet encourages chronic inflammation, without any effective means of turning it off.

Trans fatty acids add significantly to this problem. They naturally occur in very small quantities in beef (being produced in the guts of ruminants), and have traditionally played only a minor role in human diets. Over the past several decades, however, the quantity of trans fatty acids in Western diets has skyrocketed.

Partially Hydrogenated Hazards

Beginning in the 1960s and 1970s, public health officials began urging people to consume more polyunsaturated fats, particularly the omega-6 variety, and fewer saturated fats as a step toward reducing the incidence of coronary heart disease. To expand the use of omega-6 oils, food makers began hydrogenating them. Hydrogenation adds many of the qualities of saturated fat, such as butter, and also increases the amount of trans fatty acids. Until very recently, trans fatty acids were considered safe.

This is no longer the case. Scientists have learned that trans fatty acids are far more hazardous to health than are the saturated fats in butter and fatty meats. Trans fatty acids inhibit many of the enzymes needed to convert linoleic acid and alpha-linolenic acid to pro- and anti-inflammatory compounds. In essence, trans fatty acids gum up the body's processing of other fatty acids at several stages.

If all things were equal, trans fatty acids would dampen production of both the body's pro- and anti-inflammatory compounds. However, it appears that trans fatty acids inhibit more of the enzymes needed by the anti-inflammatory omega-3 fatty acids than those involved with the omega-6 fatty acids. The consequence is that trans fatty acids interfere to a greater extent with the body's anti-inflammatory compounds.

It should come as no surprise that recent studies have found trans fatty acids to significantly increase the risk of heart disease, diabetes, and other diseases. For example, a major study by Harvard University researchers found that a high intake of trans fatty acids was strongly associated with the risk of coronary heart disease. In contrast, saturated fats (commonly thought of as the culprits) were only weakly associated with heart disease.

Key Inflammation Matches and Firefighters

PRO-INFLAMMATORY MATCHES	ANTI-INFLAMMATORY FIREFIGHTERS
Linoleic acid	Alpha-linolenic acid
Vegetable oils	Gamma-linolenic acid
(e.g., corn and safflower)	Eicosapentaenoic acid (EPA)
Arachidonic acid	Oleic acid (in olive oil)
Partially hydrogenated oils	Vitamins E and C
Free radicals	

Free Radicals, Antioxidants, and Inflammation

Hazardous molecules known as free radicals damage cells and accelerate the aging process, as well as cause such age-related diseases as coronary artery disease and cancer. In simple terms free radicals lack a subatomic particle called an electron. Typically, electrons come in pairs, and to restore the pair, a free radical steals one from another molecule. That theft damages what had been a healthy cell.

Free radicals are found in virtually all dangerous chemicals, including air pollutants and cigarette smoke, and are generated when your body is exposed to radiation (even from sunlight). They are also created when your body burns food for energy, breaks down harmful chemicals in the liver, or fights infections. Indeed, your body's white blood cells generate large quantities of free radicals to destroy bacteria and virus-infected cells.

Free radicals also stimulate inflammation in several ways. They increase the activity of genes involved in making pro-inflammatory compounds such as IL-6. Free radicals also activate several different types of *adhesion molecules,* which enable various types of white blood cells to stick to other cells. Adhesion molecules should only stick to infectious microbes and damaged cells marked for cleanup. But in chronic inflammation, they can adhere to normal cells, including those in arteries and joints.

Antioxidants Are Anti-Inflammatory

The natural antidotes for free radicals are antioxidants, which include vitamins E and C and many other nutrients, particularly the many flavonoids found in vegetables, fruits, and herbs. Many antioxidants directly counteract the pro-inflammatory effects of free radicals. For example, vitamin E helps turn off genes involved in inflammation, as well as some types of adhesion molecules.

In the next chapter we will see how specific dietary changes have increased our intake of pro-inflammatory omega-6 fatty acids and decreased our consumption of anti-inflammatory omega-3 fatty acids.

CHAPTER 4

Balancing a Diet That's Out of Balance

Although imbalances in fatty acids cause much of a body's overactive inflammatory response, we need to know *why* imbalances occur. The answer is that most people no longer eat many health-promoting and anti-inflammatory foods. Instead, they eat foods that actually stoke the fires of inflammation.

Matt: Treating Multiple Sclerosis with the Original Balanced Diet

In 1995, when Matt was eighteen years old, he suddenly developed severe leg twitches, problems with balance, and an extreme sensitivity to temperature on his left side. One month later, a magnetic resonance imaging scan identified a dozen lesions in his brain and spinal column. The diagnosis was unmistakably multiple sclerosis (MS). Matt envisioned life in a wheelchair—and "almost shut down and gave up," he says.

Matt's dad, Ashton, a scientist, started reading everything about MS he could get hold of—in books, in medical journals, on the Internet. He quickly realized that few researchers and physicians had seriously considered the roles of diet and alternative treatments in controlling MS. Yet such treatments appeared to hold far more promise than drug treatments ridden with side effects.

Ashton suggested two therapies to Matt, who was initially skeptical. First came acupuncture. After ten acupuncture treatments, many of Matt's MS symptoms cleared, along with his headaches, night sweats, and allergies. Next came diet. Ashton asked Matt to follow a "Paleolithic," or caveman, diet consisting of simple and unprocessed foods such as fruits, vegetables, fish, skinless chicken breasts, and a little rice, and avoiding all dairy, gluten, legumes, fried foods, and yeast. In addition, Matt began taking a variety of supplements, including vitamins, minerals, omega-3 fatty acids, and GLA.

Since making these changes, Matt has remained completely free of MS symptoms, even while working toward his college degree and then getting a stress-filled job as a television producer. "I stick with the diet religiously," he says. "It was rough for the first six months, but then it became easy. Sure, the foods aren't real exciting, but I would rather use my hand to bring these foods to my mouth than not to be able to use my hand at all. It changed my whole perspective. I don't take as many things for granted."

Nutrients as the Building Blocks of Health

The vital role of nutrition in health is hardly a new idea. Hippocrates, who lived twenty-four hundred years ago and was the father of Western medicine, is remembered by modern physicians for the Hippocratic Oath: first, do no harm (to patients). But Hippocrates' belief that food is our best medicine is considered nothing more than quaint by many physicians familiar with it.

For many years, Western medicine has believed that therapeutic advancements are made only through science and, more recently, through technology—essentially that doctors can become masters of nature. Today, genes are considered medicine's Rosetta stone, the key to understanding why people become ill and the source of future pharmaceutical treatments. But the emphasis on genetic research and gene therapy has placed invention and technology over basic nutritional science.

There may be no better example of this folly than in genetics itself. Genes, built from molecules of deoxyribonucleic acid (DNA), certainly do contain the instructions for life. Damaged, they can and often do lead to disease. But genes do not function in a vacuum. To work the right way, genes depend on a person's consumption of the right nutrients. When genes receive inadequate nutrition or antinutrients (substances that interfere with or deplete needed nutrients), they tend to malfunction. It would be like putting water instead of gasoline in your car's fuel system.

Your body requires a variety of protein building blocks (amino acids) and some of the B-complex vitamins to make and repair DNA. In addition, many nutrients, such as vitamins C and E, protect DNA and genes from free-radical damage. Nutrients also can turn on and turn off genes, spurring them to action and calming them down. Genes may be fundamental to life, but nutrition is fundamental to genes—and all aspects of life and health.

It is essential to remember that nutrients—chiefly vitamins, minerals, proteins, and fats—are the building blocks of your entire body. They form not just your skeleton, skin, and organs, but are also the basis of your hormones and the thousands of biochemicals involved in forming new cells and tissue, healing injuries, and creating energy. Chronically low levels of nutrients or imbalances among nutrients can inhibit essential biochemical reactions and plant the seeds for degenerative diseases later in life. Yet as fundamental as nutrition is in health—and even in genetics—physicians routinely take the diets of their patients for granted. They assume that their patients are adequately nourished unless they display outright symptoms of now-rare classic vitamin deficiency diseases.

Rediscovering Our Original Diet

The huge amount of biomedical information generated in recent years has left many people confused about which diet might best enable them to thrive. How can you determine which one is the ideal—and anti-inflammatory—diet for you?

The soundest approach, in my opinion, is to study what our ancient ancestors ate and, just as importantly, what they did *not* eat. The basic idea behind the "evolutionary" diet of human beings is relatively simple. Over millions of years, humans evolved in a biological milieu that provided them certain nutrients, which became necessary for life and health. This nutritional environment helped shape our present-day genes and the rest of our biochemistry and biology.

Despite stunning cultural, scientific, and technological achievements, our genes are identical to those of Paleolithic, or Stone Age, people who lived roughly 10,000 to 40,000 years ago. Indeed, our genes have changed relatively little—only about 0.5 percent—over the 2 million previous years. We are, biologically, cavemen and cavewomen, but most of us now eat food products that did not exist until very recently.

Evolutionary vs. Modern Diets

Until relatively recently, understanding the Paleolithic diet was largely the province of anthropologists and archeologists, scientists who worked in obscurity at museums and universities. In 1985 S. Boyd Eaton, M.D., of Emory University, Atlanta, and his anthropologist colleagues published a watershed article in the *New England Journal of Medicine* that gave medical credibility to ancient nutrition.

Since that time, Eaton and his colleagues, as well as Loren Cordain, Ph.D., of Colorado State University, author of *The Paleo Diet,* have greatly expanded our understanding of the Paleolithic diet and how it differs from our modern diets. These scientists have based their ideas on a vast body of archaeological evidence, including bones, coprolites, and food remains at prehistoric sites, as well as detailed ethnographic records of 229 "hunter-gatherer" cultures that existed through the nineteenth or twentieth centuries.

Paleolithic people lived before the advent of agriculture, the intentional growing of crops. For sustenance, they hunted large and small game animals and foraged a variety of plant foods, including leaves, roots, fruits seeds, and nuts. As you might imagine, living without modern conveniences was hard and life expectancies were short, with injuries and infections being the leading causes of death. However, the archaeological record indicates that these primitive people were generally healthier than people today, and they rarely experienced our modern diseases.

It is important to note that the "typical" Paleolithic diet is a composite of many different diets, just as the average American (Western) diet also is a composite. In addition, while Paleolithic food choices varied by geography and season, they were often consistent in macronutrient (protein, carbohydrate, fat) and micronutrient (vitamin and mineral) levels, as well as in the foods *not* eaten. Despite the differences in geography, Paleolithic peoples were sophisticated hunters and gatherers, and they consumed an extraordinarily diverse selection of meats, fish (if they lived near oceans or lakes), and vegetables.

Humans Need Protein

Protein forms the foundation of our physical structure—that is, our muscle, organs, glands, and to a great extent, our bones and teeth. The components of protein are also needed by the body to synthesize DNA, hormones, neurochemicals, and other biochemicals, including those involved in pro- and anti-inflammatory reactions.

There is no evidence of an entirely vegetarian or even mostly vegetarian hunter-gatherer society. Paleolithic and hunter-gatherer societies preferred animal foods, including fish, over plant foods, according to the latest research by Cordain. Nearly three-fourths (73 percent) of hunter-gatherer societies worldwide obtained more than half of their food from animals. In contrast, only about one-eighth (14 percent) of societies obtained more than half of their food from plants. Indeed, many anthropologists believe that the development of agriculture became a necessity because human populations had overhunted large game.

The typical Paleolithic intake of protein ranged from 19 to 35 percent of calories and sometimes as much as 50 percent of calories. In general, the amount of animal foods increased and plant foods decreased in people living farther from the equator. (Long-term intake of a diet containing more than 50 percent protein can be toxic, and Cordain believes that hunter-gatherers balanced a very high protein intake by increasing their consumption of animal fat.) In contrast, the typical American adult obtains about 15 percent of his or her calories from protein, substantially less than Paleolithic peoples and hunter-gatherer societies.

Humans Need Fats

Like protein, fats have multiple roles. They help form the walls of cells and regulate what enters and exits those cells, and they also are an integral part of most all body tissues and many biochemicals. As you know, fats form the building blocks of the body's pro- and anti-inflammatory compounds.

Paleolithic people and hunter-gatherer societies consumed 28 to 58 percent of their calories in the form of fat, a quantity that is for the most part higher than the average intake of 34 percent today. Despite the large amount of fat, the specific types of fat were very different in Paleolithic times—and far more balanced in terms of inflammation-promoting or inflammation-suppressing fats. The ratio of omega-6 (inflammation-promoting) to omega-3 (inflammation-suppressing) fatty acids in the diet ranged from about 1:1 to 2:1.

Meat from wild game, the mainstay of most Paleolithic peoples and hunter-gatherer societies, is considerably leaner than meat from modern domesticated cattle. For example, grass-fed cattle (whose diet would be similar to that of wild game) have six to eight times less fat than do grain-fed cattle. In addition, beef from grass-fed cattle has two to six times more omega-3 fatty acids, compared with meat from grain-fed cattle. A similar pattern occurs in other types of livestock. Grass-fed bison have seven times more omega-3 fatty acids than do grain-fed bison. The grasses and leaves eaten by animals contain substantial amounts of omega-3 fatty acids, which are eventually deposited in the animals' muscle and fat. When people eat such meats, as they did in the past, they consume these anti-inflammatory omega-3 fatty acids.

Today's domesticated livestock are typically fed cereal grains (such as corn) for several months before slaughter, increasing their overall fat, saturated fat, and pro-inflammatory omega-6 fatty acids. Such meat contains low levels of omega-6 fatty acids and even less omega-3 fatty acids, leading to a high ratio of omega-6 to omega-3 fatty acids. For example, about 3 percent of the fat in wild game consists of omega-3 fatty acids, but only 0.4 percent (less than one-seventh the amount) of the fat in grain-fed beef does. So when people consume meat from grain-fed domesticated animals, the lopsided omega-6 to omega-3 ratio further contributes to their pro-inflammatory profile.

Perhaps surprisingly, cholesterol consumption has not changed significantly since Paleolithic times, but people now consume more of the specific saturated fats that boost the body's production of cholesterol. Elevated cholesterol levels per se are not necessarily problematic, but they can become pro-inflammatory when combined with a low intake of antioxidants, such as in a diet with few vegetables and fruit.

Based on an analysis of 829 plants, wild plant foods contain an average of 24 percent fat, a surprisingly large amount. Such plants, as well as modern leafy green vegetables (kale, spinach, dark green lettuces, greens), contain substantial amounts of alpha-linolenic acid, the building block of the omega-3 fatty acids. During our evolutionary development this mix of natural, uncultivated plant foods and wild game meat led to a balanced intake of omega-6 and omega-3 fatty acids, which tempered abnormal inflammatory responses.

Especially significant, Paleolithic peoples and later hunter-gatherer societies did not consume *any* oils or fats unless they were part of meat or vegetables. Our ancestors *never* consumed pressed or refined oils. This contrasts sharply with today, with corn, soy, and safflower oil—all rich in pro-inflammatory omega-6 fatty acids—being ubiquitous in kitchens and foods. These oils, often manipulated to mimic saturated fats and to form trans fatty acids, are used to lubricate fry pans; to deep-fry potatoes, chicken, and fish; and are added to the vast majority of processed (packaged) foods, such as salad dressings, microwave meals, meat extenders, baked goods, and chocolate bars.

Switching from a diet high in saturated fat to one high in omega-6 fatty acids—the very change that public health authorities have recommended to Americans over the past thirty years—actually decreases the body's production of anti-inflammatory omega-3 compounds (specifically, EPA and DHA) by 40 to 50 percent. In addition, many foods, such as fried potatoes and fried chicken, are cooked in oxidized vegetable oils, increasing their content of free radicals and adding to the pro-inflammatory burden.

Humans Need Carbohydrates and Fiber

Carbohydrates, made up of starches and sugars, provide most of the body's energy—that is, they are burned for fuel or stored as fat. In Paleolithic times and in hunter-gatherer societies, carbohydrates came almost entirely from uncultivated low-starch vegetables (leaves, shoots, buds, roots), fruit, seeds, and nuts. The carbohydrates in uncultivated and unprocessed vegetables are complex, meaning that they are digested slowly, in contrast to simple sugars, which are absorbed rapidly. Complex carbohydrates are part of the plant's matrix, which includes substantial amounts of protein, vitamins, minerals, and indigestible fiber. In other words, Paleolithic peoples and hunter-gatherer societies ate relatively low-carbohydrate diets, and the carbohydrates were not readily absorbed.

Today, only a minority of people regularly consume substantive amounts of vegetables and fruit daily. Instead, the vast majority of dietary carbohydrates and calories come from highly refined grains (chiefly wheat but also corn and rye), sugars (sucrose and high-fructose corn syrup, particularly in soft drinks and other beverages), and fried potatoes (which contain trans fatty acids and oxidized omega-6 fatty acids).

One excellent marker of vegetable intake is dietary fiber content. In Paleolithic times, people ate an average of 100 grams of fiber daily, almost entirely from vegetables and fruit. Today, the typical Westerner eats only 20 grams daily, mostly from grains. Although whole grains, such as whole-wheat bread, provide some vitamins, minerals, and fiber, they still fall far short of vegetables in vitamins, minerals, and fiber. And as grain consumption has increased over the years, vegetable and fruit consumption has decreased.

The impact of refined grains and sugars on inflammation is significant, though not as obvious as with oils and fats. Consumption of refined grains and sugars typically raises blood sugar levels and, over the long term, increases the risk of diabetes. Recently, researchers have reported that very modest chronic increases in blood sugar, even when in the normal range, significantly increase the risk of developing diabetes or heart disease within just a few years. Both diseases have inflammatory undercurrents, and elevations in blood sugar spontaneously generate free radicals, which can stimulate inflammation.

Humans Need Vitamins, Minerals, and Phytonutrients

Over the course of a year Paleolithic peoples and hunter-gatherer societies typically consumed more than a hundred different types of plants. These were very different foods from what most people consume today. Ancient uncultivated vegetables were more akin to nutrient-packed kale than to iceberg lettuce, and uncultivated fruit looked more like crabapples and rose hips than supersweet pears and bananas.

Only 9 to 32 percent of North Americans consume the five daily servings of vegetables and fruit recommended by the federal government, meaning that 68 to 91 percent of Americans do not eat a particularly rich dietary source of vitamins and other micronutrients. Of those people who do eat vegetables and fruit, most choose from a limited selection, such as potatoes, which are often fried; corn; peas; carrots; and iceberg lettuce. As a consequence, most people today fall far short of the greater quantity and diversity of vitamins, minerals, and phytonutrients consumed by Paleolithic peoples and hunter-gatherers.

Based on the calculations by Eaton and Cordain, Paleolithic peoples consumed an average of two to ten times more vitamins and minerals than people do today. These levels range from three to six times the federal government's Recommended Dietary Allowance (or Daily Value) for vitamins and minerals. For example, a Paleolithic person likely ate about 600 mg of vitamin C daily, compared with an RDA of 60 mg, and a typical North American daily intake of 45 mg or less daily.

In addition, vegetables and fruit contain large amounts of vitaminlike antioxidant nutrients, particularly flavonoids and carotenoids. A diet containing a diverse selection of vegetables and fruit would likely provide hundreds of flavonoids and dozens of carotenoids. Researchers estimate that people nowadays consume between 23 and 170 mg of flavonoids daily, but that they may have consumed five to twenty-four times more (115 to 4,080 mg daily) in the past. Such a huge dietary intake of antioxidants—now missing from most people's diets—would moderate inflammatory reactions.

—☓—

Past and Present Intake of Vitamins and Minerals

VITAMINS	PALEOLITHIC* (MG/DAY)	CURRENT U.S.† (MG/DAY)	RATIO
Vitamin C	604	93	6.5
Vitamin E	32.8	8.5	3.9
Vitamin B₂	6.49	1.71	3.8
Vitamin B₁	3.91	1.42	2.8
Vitamin A	17.2	7.8	2.2
Folic acid	0.36	0.18	2

MINERALS	PALEOLITHIC* (MG/DAY)	CURRENT U.S.† (MG/DAY)	RATIO
Copper	12.2	1.2	10.2
Iron	87.4	10.5	8.3
Manganese	13.3	3	4.4
Potassium	10,500	2,500	4.2
Magnesium	1,223	320	3.8
Zinc	43.4	12.5	3.5
Phosphorus	3,223	1,510	2.1
Calcium	1,622	920	1.8
Sodium	768	4,000	0.2

* Based on 3,000 calories daily, 35 percent animal and 65 percent plant subsistence.
† Average of U.S. men and women; Food and Nutrition Board, 1989.

—☓—

The Turning Points in Our Diet

Americans, and increasingly Canadians and Europeans, certainly do enjoy full stomachs. The latest statistics show that 65 percent of Americans (two of every three) are overweight and 31 percent (almost one in three) are clinically obese—at least thirty pounds over their ideal weight. Being overweight is not a sign of good nutrition; rather, it is a sign of excessive calorie and carbohydrate intake, usually at the expense of more nutrient-dense and wholesome foods.

There are many ways to look at the history of dietary changes and to analyze how these changes have affected people's health. Because this book is about inflammation, the emphasis in our brief examination of food history will be on how the diet has shifted from relatively balanced to clearly pro-inflammatory. Three major periods of dietary change have occurred: the agricultural revolution, the industrial revolution, and the convenience/fast-food revolution. All of these changes have been characterized by two basic trends: (1) through a variety of processing and refining methods, the modern diet less and less resembles our evolutionary diet, and (2) the majority of foods sold in supermarkets less and less resemble their original appearance in nature.

—〽—

How the Diet Has Changed

PALEOLITHIC DIET

Highly diverse diet, consisting of lean meats, fish, and vegetable matter

Balanced intake (1:1 ratio) of pro- and anti-inflammatory fats and very high intake of anti-inflammatory vitamins and minerals

AGRICULTURAL REVOLUTION

Greatly increased intake of grains, lower intake of vegetables and meat

Displacement of nutrient-dense vegetables and meat with moderate shift toward pro-inflammatory diet

INDUSTRIAL REVOLUTION

Extensive refining and processing of grains and sugar, enabling large segments of the population to afford and consume such foods

Further displacement of nutrient-dense foods and greater risk of elevated pro-inflammatory blood sugar levels

CONVENIENCE/FAST-FOOD REVOLUTION

Refining, processing, and industrial manipulation of foods widespread, creating a typical diet high in carbohydrates, unbalanced fat intake, and very low intake of vegetables

Diet contains twenty to thirty times more pro-inflammatory than anti-inflammatory fats and substantially fewer anti-inflammatory vitamins and minerals

—〽—

The Agricultural Revolution

The first major changes to the diet—that is, departures from lean meat, fish, and plant foods—occurred approximately ten thousand years ago with the development of agriculture, the domestication of livestock, and the use of milk and other dairy products. Agriculture stabilized the movement of hunter-gatherer societies, which eventually led to the growth of cities and the development of complex cultures. But the use of grains also led to health problems that were not immediately evident.

The cultivation and consumption of grains introduced the protein gluten to the diet of humans. Gluten is an umbrella term for forty related proteins in a handful of grains, particularly wheat, rye, and barley. You might think that a new vegetarian source of protein would be good, but gluten has been a mixed blessing.

Many people—approximately one in every hundred—are allergic to gluten, causing what is known as celiac disease. In these people, eating gluten triggers an immune (inflammatory) response, which primarily attacks the gastrointestinal tract and interferes with vitamin and mineral absorption. Archeologists have noted that the health of humans, based largely on analysis of ancient bones, took a turn for the worse after gluten-containing grains became popular foods. Osteoporosis, arthritis, and even birth defects became more common after people began eating grains.

The health effects of gluten proteins in grains may be problematic for many people who do not have an inborn sensitivity to gluten. According to Melissa Diane Smith, a nutritionist and author of *Going Against the Grain,* half of Westerners may be sensitive to gluten without exhibiting any of the traditional symptoms of celiac disease. Instead, gluten sensitivity may appear as immunological reactions affecting the nervous system, balance, and behavior, as well as a person's overall sense of well-being. According to Smith, a second family of grain (and legume) proteins, called lectins, may also damage the gut and interfere with nutrient absorption. Meanwhile, Loren Cordain's research has shown that lectins play a role in rheumatoid arthritis and possibly other inflammatory autoimmune diseases. The bottom line is that most grains are neither the much-heralded staff of life nor the breakfast of champions.

Ten millennia ago—too short of a time for genetic evolution—people also began domesticating livestock for meat and, in the case of cows and goats, for milk and other dairy products. As long as livestock were exclusively grass-fed, their meat and milk yielded a balance of pro- and anti-inflammatory fatty acids. This changed when animals were fed corn,

—⚡—

Some Differences between Paleolithic and Modern Diets

	PALEOLITHIC	MODERN
FOOD GROUP		
Protein	Very lean	Fatty
Carbohydrates	From vegetables	From grains and refined sugars
Fats	Balanced intake	Pro-inflammatory
FOOD TYPES		
Animal/fish foods*	65 percent of diet	15 percent of diet
Vegetables/fruit	About 100 different plants	Very narrow selection
Fiber	100 grams daily	20 grams daily
Vitamins/minerals	Substantially more	Substantially less
Grains	None	Substantial intake
Dairy	None	Substantial intake
Pressed oils	None	Substantial intake
Trans fatty acids	Negligible	Substantial intake
Alcohol	None	3 percent of calories

* Animal and fish foods were not exclusively protein. These foods also supplied fat and bone.

—⚡—

which, as previously noted, increases the animals' overall fat and saturated fat and reduces anti-inflammatory omega-3 fatty acids.

Many people have questioned the health benefits of cow's milk, but a couple of points are especially relevant in the context of our evolutionary diet. One is that no species, other than humans over the past ten thousand years, has ever consumed milk beyond infancy. Another is that no species other than humans has ever consumed the milk of another mammal. Like grains, cow's milk appears to be a mismatch for our genetic heritage. The situation is made worse today because milk products from grain-fed cows contain no appreciable amounts of omega-3 fatty acids.

The Industrial Revolution

Many dietary changes occurred over the next ten millennia, including greater cultivation of vegetables and fruit, which increased the sugar content and reduced the bitterness of produce. But perhaps the most significant changes relate to the refining of wheat, which has become a staple food. The use of new technologies to refine grains as well as sugars foreshadowed many other changes.

In the nineteenth century metal rollers replaced stone grinding wheels (grindstones), enabling millers to achieve a more mechanized and efficient means of processing grains into flour. Grains could be processed faster, yielding much finer flour, without bits of stone being eroded and ending up in the flour. In addition, the new technologies enabled easier separation of the grain's germ and bran from the endosperm, which was mostly carbohydrate. The nutrient-lacking endosperm was used for baking bread and other products, whereas the germ and bran were often fed to livestock. In addition, the endosperm-based flour used in baking was bleached chemically to make it white, increasing its consumer appeal.

The industrialization of the grain-refining process yielded "white bread" for the masses instead of only for a limited number of wealthy people. Nutritionally, the difference between whole-grain and white bread was disastrous. During the 1930s increasing consumption of white bread contributed to deficiencies of several B vitamins in North America and Europe. The situation led to government-mandated "enrichment" of flours to replace a handful of the many nutrients removed during grain refining.

The Convenience/Fast-Food Revolution

After the end of World War II, technologists helped guide unprecedented prosperity in the United States. The first Swanson brand TV dinner, a frozen meal on a metal tray, was introduced in 1953, heralding the start of the convenience/fast-food revolution. It was a commercial success. Several years later, in southern California, automobiles and food intersected, giving birth to McDonald's and the fast-food industry. The trade-off for fast, convenient food was lower nutritional value and fewer anti-inflammatory nutrients.

Meanwhile, more women entered the workforce and had less time than before to prepare large home-cooked meals—with most men not helping. The need to reduce time in the kitchen fueled the popularity of the microwave oven in the 1970s. TV dinners that baked in the oven for forty minutes were quickly replaced by microwave meals ready in fewer than five minutes. For the first time in history, large numbers of people did not have to wait very long, or expend much effort, before sitting down and eating. This was a major change from when people spent their entire days hunting and gathering food.

The economic climate of the 1990s reinforced the demand for convenience and fast—and faster—food. The entire pace of business quickened with the pressures of international competition, overnight deliveries, and e-mail. People who had once comfortably ended their workday at 5:00 P.M. are now connected to their offices 24/7 via e-mail, pagers, and cell phones. More and more, fast and convenience foods have become the way to sandwich meals into hectic schedules.

For the most part, these meals are made with ingredients high in refined carbohydrates and pro-inflammatory omega-6 and trans fatty acids and very low in vitamins, minerals, fiber, and protein. A recent study published in the *Journal of the American Dietetic Association* found that two-thirds of the carbohydrates consumed by American adults come from bread, soft drinks, cakes and cookies, refined cereal, pasta, cooked grains, and ice cream. These refined carbohydrates raise blood sugar levels, creating a prediabetic or diabeticlike blood profile, which generates pro-inflammatory free radicals. Recent research by Simin Liu, M.D., Ph.D., of Harvard Medical School has found that diets high in refined carbohydrates and high-glycemic foods (which rapidly raise blood sugar levels) increase inflammation. In Liu's study, women eating large amounts of potatoes, breakfast cereals, white bread, muffins, and white rice had elevated C-reactive protein levels, indicating high levels of inflammation and an increased risk of heart disease. Overweight women who ate a lot of these foods had the highest and most dangerous CRP levels. All of these carbohydrates (and the fat they are often combined with) displace far healthier foods, such as anti-inflammatory vegetables, fruit, and fish.

In addition, research published in November 2002 showed that yet another inflammation-causing substance forms when foods are cooked at high temperatures. Advanced glycation end products (AGEs) are created when sugars bind in a particular way to proteins. As the acronym suggests, AGEs accelerate the aging process. However, AGEs also increase levels of C-reactive protein, a powerful promoter of inflammation. In a study with diabetic patients, those who consumed foods cooked at high temperatures had a 65 percent increase in AGEs after just two weeks. However, people eating the same foods cooked at low temperatures had a 30 percent decrease in AGEs. The AGE-lowering foods were cooked by boiling or steaming—or were quickly sautéed with a small amount of oil. Baking foods for hours, such as how the typical Thanksgiving turkey is prepared, generates large amounts of AGEs. In addition, coffee, cola drinks, chocolate drinks, and fried foods are very high in AGEs.

—⚏—

A New Definition of Hot and Cold Foods

It helps to look at foods as either "hot" pro-inflammatory or "cold" anti-inflammatory. Hot foods set the stage for the burning pain of inflammation, whereas cold foods reduce inflammation.

"HOT" PRO-INFLAMMATORY FOODS	"COLD" ANTI-INFLAMMATORY FOODS
Most vegetable oils	Olive oil
French fries	Fish, particularly cold-water
Fried chicken and fish	species
Margarine	Fresh vegetables
Most salad dressings	Low-sugar fruits (e.g., berries)
Breads and other bakery products	Free-range beef and chicken
Many packaged microwave foods	Game meats (not corn-fed)
Fast-food meals	Mineral water
Beverages with sugars	

—⚏—

What is the bottom line with all of these refined, processed foods? First, they displace many important nutrients, such as anti-inflammatory vitamins, minerals, protein, and omega-3 fatty acids. Second, many grains contain antinutrients, which actually interfere with normal nutrient absorption. Third, highly refined sugars and carbohydrates draw nutrients such as vitamins and minerals from the body's reserves to aid the metabolic processes that normally burn these foods for energy. Fourth, the sheer quantity of calories and carbohydrates in refined sugars and carbohydrates promotes obesity, and fat cells generate large quantities of interleukin-6 and C-reactive protein, two of the most powerful pro-inflammatory compounds made by the body.

The end result is a diet high in pro-inflammatory fats, devoid of anti-inflammatory fats, and nearly empty of anti-inflammatory antioxidants.

And anti-inflammatory drugs don't really help, as we'll see in the next chapter.

CHAPTER 5

What's Wrong with Anti-Inflammatory Drugs

Melinda: When the Cure Is Worse Than the Disease

You might think that "iatrogenic disease" is some sort of rare condition. But the term actually refers to any illness caused by a physician or treatment. And it's surprisingly common. In a typical year, more than a hundred thousand hospitalized patients die from medications they had been prescribed, and more than 2 million others suffer severe side effects. Incredibly, no one knows the number of serious adverse reactions and deaths from drugs related to over-the-counter medications.

When Melinda was in her midthirties, she sought more aggressive medical treatment of her allergies and asthma, as well as of her increasingly stiff joints. Up to this point, she had used either over-the-counter or prescription antihistamines for her allergies, nasal corticosteroid hormones for her asthma, and ibuprofen (an NSAID, or nonsteroidal anti-inflammatory drug) for her rheumatoid arthritis.

Melinda's physician put her on prednisone, a hormone treatment for allergies and arthritis, and a potent prescription-strength NSAID. Side effects from the prednisone included a seventy-pound weight gain, weakened bones, and increased susceptibility to colds and flus, which left

Melinda feeling tired much of the time. The NSAID caused a painful gastric ulcer, which was treated by a drug to reduce stomach acid.

The medications and Melinda's weight gain substantially increased her risk of heart disease and, particularly, heart failure (a catastrophic weakening of the heart muscle). Melinda's physician tried to head off the damage, but he relied solely on pharmaceutical treatment and never discussed nutrition or an anti-inflammatory diet with her. Two years later, after a battery of laboratory tests, he noted that her C-reactive protein levels were elevated, a sign of serious inflammation, so he prescribed a cholesterol-lowering "statin" drug to reduce her risk of heart disease.

The statin drug lowered Melinda's cholesterol, but it also reduced her body's production of coenzyme Q_{10}, a vitaminlike substance needed for normal heart function. Both the statin and the NSAID increased her risk of heart failure. As Melinda's heart function declined, her physician prescribed one more drug to stimulate the heart.

Sadly, her downward spiral could not be stopped. Melinda died of heart failure at age thirty-nine, even though her symptoms could have been reversed by diet and safe nutritional supplements.

With dozens of over-the-counter and prescription anti-inflammatory drugs on the market, you might think that the cure for your aches and pains is as near as the corner pharmacy. Many of these drugs, such as aspirin and ibuprofen, provide relief to millions of people around the world. But these and other drugs have a dark side that, perhaps in the majority of cases, outweighs their benefits. In this chapter we will look at the hazards of several classes of anti-inflammatory drugs.

Anti-Inflammatory Drugs and Their Hazards

Pharmaceutical drugs, used appropriately and for short periods of time, can quickly relieve pain and inflammation. However, they are anything but magic bullets. The longer such drugs are used, and this is the case with chronic inflammatory diseases, the greater the risk of serious side effects.

Drug companies market more than 30 different types of NSAIDs, the most widely used class of drugs. Many other drugs also are used to treat inflammation, and 250 are sold for the treatment of arthritis alone. Each year, pharmacists in the United States fill more than 70 million prescriptions for NSAIDs, and consumers buy about 30 billion over-the-counter

NSAID products. According to an article in the *New England Journal of Medicine,* NSAID complications lead to 7,500 bleeding ulcers, 103,000 hospitalizations, and 16,500 deaths annually (about the same number of deaths caused by AIDS), costing more than $2 billion in medical expenses.

Three classes of medications are used to treat inflammatory diseases, and a fourth is rapidly emerging. These medications are corticosteroids, conventional over-the-counter and prescription NSAIDs, the first generation of selective Cox-2 inhibiting NSAIDs, and the relatively new use of "statin" drugs to reduce C-reactive protein levels.

Corticosteroids

Introduced in the 1950s, cortisonelike drugs called corticosteroids or glucocorticoids became—and still are—extraordinarily popular. These drugs are synthetic mimics of stress-response hormones produced in the adrenal glands. Physicians can choose among dozens of corticosteroids to treat inflammation, but perhaps the best-known corticosteroid is prednisone, which is sold under a variety of brand names.

Corticosteroids are frequently the first treatment physicians prescribe to patients diagnosed with autoimmune diseases such as rheumatoid arthritis, asthma, lupus erythematosus, or multiple sclerosis. They rapidly and dramatically dampen the body's overactive immune response and sometimes are necessary as a *brief* intervention. That's the good news. The bad news about prednisone and other corticosteroids reads like a chamber of medical horrors. Over several weeks or months, oral or injected corticosteroids affect almost every organ and lead to serious side effects while the drugs are being taken, as well as permanent damage.

Among the most common side effects is a rounded "moon face," which is considered characteristic of prednisone use. An increase in abdominal obesity also is common. Because prednisone and other corticosteroids dampen the immune response, they increase susceptibility to infection, often masking symptoms of active infections, and they interfere with the normal healing of wounds. As a consequence, people taking corticosteroids for many weeks or months are more susceptible to infections; and cuts, scrapes, and more serious injuries are slow to heal.

Corticosteroids also interfere with the metabolism of key nutrients, including folic acid, vitamins B_6 and B_{12}, potassium, and zinc. Because these drugs also reduce vitamin D and calcium levels, they prevent normal bone development in young people. In adults, long-term use of corticosteroids leads to decreased bone density and osteoporosis. Some corticosteroids can be injected directly into the joints of people with arthritis, but repeated injections accelerate joint damage.

Other common side effects of corticosteroids include a thinning of the skin and bruising, high blood pressure, elevated blood sugar levels (which increase the risk of diabetes and coronary artery disease), cataracts and glaucoma, male infertility, menstrual irregularities, and loss of muscle mass.

Conventional NSAIDs

Aspirin, ibuprofen (Advil, Motrin, and generic brands), naproxen sodium, (Aleve and others) are the most popular over-the-counter nonsteroidal anti-inflammatory drugs, and many higher-potency NSAIDs are available by prescription. The term NSAID means that these drugs are anti-inflammatory but not based on steroid hormones. NSAIDs are very effective in relieving headaches, controlling inflammation, easing pain, and reducing fevers. But like other anti-inflammatory drugs, they pose considerable dangers, particularly when used regularly.

Aspirin, which has been widely used since about 1900, is the oldest pharmaceutical NSAID. Before aspirin was synthesized, people often used willow bark, which contains a compound very similar to synthetic aspirin. For many years, researchers believed that NSAIDs worked by inhibiting the activity of cyclooxygenase, an enzyme critical to the conversion of fatty acids to pro- and anti-inflammatory compounds. In the early 1990s researchers discovered a second form of cyclooxygenase, so the two compounds are now referred to as Cox-1 and Cox-2. The prevailing view in medicine has been that Cox-1, whose levels are generally steady, performs normal cell functions. In contrast, doctors have believed that Cox-2 levels rise as part of the body's inflammatory response.

In the course of research scientists quickly realized that most NSAIDs interfere with both Cox-1 and Cox-2, causing a variety of side effects in many people. The most common side effect of NSAIDs is an upset stomach, which affects at least 10 to 20 percent of people taking these drugs, but according to some studies may affect up to 50 percent. In 10 to 25 percent of people regularly taking NSAIDs, the stomach wall erodes, leading to gastritis (inflammation of the stomach wall) and the formation of gastric ulcers. Ironically, as physicians have successfully treated *Helicobacter pylori* infections, a major cause of stomach ulcers, NSAIDs have become the leading cause of ulcers. The reason is NSAIDs' suppression of Cox-1, which is essential for maintaining the integrity of stomach and duodenal (upper part of the intestine, just below the stomach) walls.

NSAID-induced damage to the gut wall can lead to leaky-gut syndrome. A leaky gut increases the permeability of the stomach wall and permits incompletely digested proteins to enter the bloodstream, where they can trigger inflammatory immune reactions. Allergylike food sensitivities, whether inborn or caused by a leaky gut, can worsen pollen allergies, and they have been shown to increase symptoms of rheumatoid arthritis. Indeed, the "feel better one day, feel worse another day" nature of osteoarthritis and rheumatoid arthritis may reflect sporadic exposure to food allergens.

Aspirin, specifically, also is a potent anticoagulant, largely because it interferes with chemicals involved in blood clotting. Many physicians recommend a very small amount of aspirin daily to reduce the long-term risk of coronary artery disease. But aspirin's blood-thinning effect also increases the tendency toward bleeding (such as in nosebleeds) and bleeding time, making wounds slower to close and heal.

Two lines of research indicate that NSAIDs can be even more dangerous. A recent study published in *Archives of Internal Medicine* found that the regular use of NSAIDs (other than aspirin) doubles a person's risk of being hospitalized for heart failure. Physicians John Page, M.B.B.S., and David Henry M.B.ChB., of the University of Newcastle, Newcastle, Australia, found that NSAID use among seniors with a history of heart disease increased the risk of hospitalization for heart failure by ten times. Seniors are the biggest users of NSAIDs, chiefly for rheumatoid arthritis, osteoarthritis, and other aches and pains. Page and Henry calculated that NSAID use might account for 19 percent (almost one-fifth) of all hospital admissions for heart failure, one of the most serious of all heart diseases.

The other, truly mind-boggling feature of regular NSAID use is that some of these drugs, particularly aspirin and ibuprofen, have been to shown to *accelerate* the breakdown of cartilage in joints. This is especially ironic among people who take NSAIDs to relieve the pain of osteoarthritis, a disease characterized by the destruction of cartilage padding in the joints. Although this breakdown of joint cartilage is very well documented, few patients are ever told of it. In a perverse irony the use of NSAIDs to relieve osteoarthritic pain actually speeds up the underlying disease process. (Although acetaminophen is not an NSAID, it appears to have a similar effect on promoting osteoarthritis.)

Cox-2 Inhibitors

With the discovery of two forms of cyclooxygenase, and the belief that only Cox-2 was involved in inflammation, several pharmaceutical companies began massive research projects to develop a new generation of Cox-2 inhibitors. In theory, these drugs would stop inflammation by suppressing Cox-2 activity, but avoid gastrointestinal side effects associated with inhibition of Cox-1.

Celebrex and Vioxx were the first "selective" Cox-2 inhibitors. But the new generation of Cox-2 inhibitors (often referred to as "coxibs") was only 20 percent selective for Cox-2. In other words they were 80 percent, just like traditional NSAIDs. Coxibs were no more effective therapeutically and no safer than earlier NSAIDs.

One study, testing Vioxx against naproxen, found that the Cox-2 inhibitor increased the incidence of heart attack by four times, compared with the older NSAID. A recent analysis of four studies of Cox-2 inhibitors confirmed that this new class of drugs increases the risk of heart attack and stroke, according to an article in the *Journal of the American Medical Association.*

The problems run even deeper. The drug companies assumed that only Cox-2, not Cox-1, was involved in inflammatory reactions. It now appears that both Cox-1 and Cox-2 play fundamental housekeeping roles in cells and normal health, and both also have roles in inflammation. In other words the very theory behind the development of selective coxibs may well have been wrong.

Researchers have recently discovered that Cox-2 has diverse fundamental roles in human biology, aside from its place in eicosanoid production. Like Cox-1, Cox-2 is involved in maintaining the integrity of the stomach wall, as well as in normal kidney and blood platelet function. Cox-2 also appears to be active in brain development, activity, and memory. It also is involved in ovulation and implantation of the egg into the womb. So it should come as no surprise that suppression of Cox-2 leads to undesirable side effects. It is likely that other undesirable side effects will emerge after the second generation of Cox-2 inhibitors reach the marketplace.

CRP-Lowering Agents

C-reactive protein (CRP) has long been recognized as an indicator of intense, systemic (bodywide) inflammation. Slowly, experts have come to see CRP as a promoter of inflammation, instead of simply as a marker.

In the late 1990s Paul M. Ridker, M.D., of Harvard Medical School, found that elevated blood levels of CRP increased the risk of heart attack by 4.5 times, a relationship far stronger than that between cholesterol or homocysteine and heart disease. Other research teams have found that elevated CRP levels are associated with Alzheimer's, arthritis, cancer, diabetes, overweight, asthma, and many other inflammatory diseases. The body makes CRP from interleukin-6, one of the most pro-inflammatory of all cytokines. Although some CRP is made in the liver, an organ best described as the body's chemical processing factor, large amounts also are made by abdominal fat cells.

Although many studies have found that vitamin E and other nutrients significantly reduce CRP levels, several major pharmaceutical trials have begun positioning "statin" drugs as the therapy of choice for lowering CRP levels. The statin drugs, which include Lipitor (atorvastatin), Mevacor (lovastatin), Pravachol (pravastatin), Zocor (simvastatin), Baycol (cerivastatin), and the more recent Bextra (valdecoxib), have been the most common medical treatments for lowering cholesterol.

Despite their popularity and a common perception of safety, statins pose serious risks. They reduce the body's production of cholesterol by inhibiting an enzyme known as HMG-CoA-reductase. This enzyme is active early in a series of biochemical reactions that eventually leads to the production of cholesterol (which, by the way, is the core molecule in all of the body's steroid hormones, including estrogen, testosterone, and corticosteroids). The problem is that statins also turn off the body's production of all the other compounds that depend on HMG-CoA-reductase.

One of these downstream compounds is coenzyme Q_{10} (CoQ_{10}). CoQ_{10} is a vitaminlike substance that plays a pivotal role in how the body's cells produce energy. CoQ_{10} is so crucial to health that research on it formed the basis of the 1978 Nobel Prize in chemistry. A small number of cardiologists in the United States and Europe, and far more in Japan, have successfully used large amounts (approximately 400 mg daily) of supplemental CoQ_{10} to treat cardiomyopathy and heart failure, diseases characterized by a catastrophic loss of energy in heart cells.

All of these findings should raise red flags about the use of statins in lowering cholesterol and, now, in lowering CRP levels. One common side effect of statins is muscle weakness, significant because muscle cells (particularly the heart) contain the largest amounts of CoQ_{10}. In August 2001 Bayer A.G., a giant German pharmaceutical company, withdrew its Baycol statin drug from the marketplace. Thirty-one patients had died while taking the drug, all because of a rare condition in which muscle tissue broke down.

Although anti-inflammatory drugs can be therapeutically useful at times, they treat symptoms and not the causes of disease, and some even speed the progression of inflammatory diseases. The side effects of anti-inflammatory drugs derive from the fact that they are biochemical interlopers that disrupt, rather than enhance, the normal functions of the body.

In the next chapter and the remainder of this book we will focus on safe dietary changes and supplements to boost the body's production of natural anti-inflammatory substances.

PART II

The Anti-Inflammation Syndrome Diet Plan

CHAPTER 6

Fifteen Steps to Fight the Inflammation Syndrome

—ₘ—

QUIZ 2

What Are Your Current Eating Habits?

Rationale: Highly processed foods—those most commonly eaten—contain many pro-inflammatory substances. If you are not very careful about what you eat, you likely consume large amounts of pro-inflammatory foods.

Eating Habits at Home

Do you or your significant other cook with corn, peanut, sunflower, safflower, or soy oil (as opposed to olive or grapeseed oil)?

Add 3 points _____

Do you eat a prepackaged microwave meal that provides a full meal (as opposed to only frozen vegetables) more than once a week?

Add 1 point _____

Do you eat any foods packaged in boxes, such as ready-to-eat cereals, flavored rices, meat extenders, and other boxed foods, more than once a week?

Add 1 point _____

When you eat at home, do you use bottled salad dressings that contain soy or safflower oil or partially hydrogenated fats (as opposed to olive oil)? Check the label.

Add 2 points _____

Do you eat pasta, bread, or pizza (one, some, or all three) daily?

Add 2 points _____

Do you eat baked goods, such as cookies, coffee cakes, other cakes, doughnuts, packaged brownies, cakes, or similar food products at least once a week?

Add 2 points _____

Do you use margarine instead of butter?

Add 2 points _____

Do you eat a lot of hamburgers?

Add 1 point _____

Do you dislike eating fish?

Add 1 point _____

Do you drink regular (sweetened) soft drinks or add sugar to your coffee or tea?

Add 1 point _____

Eating Habits in Restaurants

Do you eat at fast-food restaurants such as McDonald's, Burger King, KFC, Taco Bell, or others at least once a week?

Add 2 points _____

Do you eat at a Chinese restaurant more than once a week?

Add 2 points _____

Do you eat pasta or pizza in a restaurant at least once a week?

Add 2 points _____

Do you eat breaded and fried fish or deep-fried shrimp more than once every week or two?

Add 2 points _____

Do you eat French fries?

Add 2 points _____

Do you eat mostly beef?

Add 1 point _____

If you eat beef, is hamburger your favorite type?

Add 1 point _____

Do you order soft drinks when you eat out?

Add 1 point _____

Your score on quiz 2: _____

Interpretation and ranking:

- **0–2 Low.** You are eating a low-inflammation diet, which is the best way to protect yourself from chronic inflammation.
- **3–5 Moderate.** You are eating a moderate-inflammation diet, which may set the stage for chronic inflammation.
- **6–19 High.** You are eating a high-inflammation diet, which substantially increases your risk of inflammatory diseases.
- **20+ Very high.** You are eating a very high inflammation diet, which greatly increases your risk of disease.

High or very high on quiz 2 but not quiz 1 (page 14): You are at risk for developing inflammatory diseases in the coming years. This would be a good time to bolster your long-term health.

High or very high on both *quiz 1 and quiz 2:* You likely have a high level of inflammation. The reason is probably that you are eating too many pro-inflammatory foods. You would do well to go on the Anti-Inflammation Syndrome Diet Plan and take steps to improve your long-term health.

High or very high on quiz 1 but not quiz 2: You have probably adopted a very good diet but may have to further fine-tune your diet and supplement program.

—⟋⟍—

Now that you understand how the modern diet sets the stage for abnormally strong inflammatory reactions, you can focus on eating anti-inflammatory and neutral foods. The best anti-inflammatory foods are fish, especially cold-water varieties such as salmon, and a diverse selection of vegetables. The old adage "Eat a lot of color" definitely applies here because, to a great extent, bright and deep colors often indicate the presence of natural anti-inflammatory nutrients.

In this chapter you will read about fifteen anti-inflammation dietary steps to follow while cooking at home or eating out. These steps form the foundation of the Anti-Inflammation Syndrome Diet Plan. Don't worry about trying to remember all fifteen of the steps. If you adhere strictly to step 1, you won't have to remember most of the remaining ones, and following just some of the steps will likely be a major improvement over your current diet. The fifteenth step adapts the Anti-Inflammation Syndrome Diet Plan for losing weight, so it may or may not apply to you. Maintaining a normal weight is important because fat increases the amount of inflammation-causing substances made by the body.

Although the steps are remarkably simple, some may seem difficult to follow at the beginning, because you will have to break some bad eating habits and learn some good ones. It is important to remember that your previous eating habits created health problems for you, and that fact should help motivate you to stick with your new eating habits. If you still dread making these changes, give them a try for just one week. You will likely start to feel noticeably better during this time.

The goals of the Anti-Inflammation Syndrome Diet Plan are twofold: one, offsetting the damage of a pro-inflammatory diet, and two, restoring and maintaining a diet that reduces your risk of chronic inflammatory diseases and symptoms. By emphasizing anti-inflammatory foods, at least for several months, you can establish a more normal balance between pro- and anti-inflammatory compounds in your body. Once you have achieved such a balance, you may be able to eat more "neutral" foods and even tolerate an occasional pro-inflammatory food.

You will be pleased to know that the Anti-Inflammation Syndrome Diet Plan does not ask that you eat like a caveman or a cavewoman—but it does encourage you to take the best of the past and current knowledge of nutrition science. As you will discover when trying the recipes in the following chapter, the diet is relatively easy and tasty.

—◊◊◊—

The Anti-Inflammation Syndrome Diet Steps

1. Eat a variety of fresh and whole foods.
2. Eat more fish, especially cold-water varieties.
3. Eat lean meats (not corn-fed) from free-range chicken and turkey, grass-fed cattle and buffalo, and game meats such as duck and ostrich.
4. Eat a lot of vegetables, the more colorful the better.
5. Use spices and herbs to flavor foods, and limit your use of salt and pepper.
6. Use olive oil as your primary cooking oil.

7. Avoid conventional cooking oils such as corn, safflower, sunflower, and soybean oil, as well as vegetable shortening, margarine, and partially hydrogenated oils.
8. Identify and avoid food allergens.
9. Avoid or strictly limit your intake of food products that contain sugars, such as sucrose or high-fructose corn syrup.
10. Avoid or limit your intake of refined grains.
11. Limit your intake of dairy products.
12. Snack on nuts and seeds.
13. When thirsty, drink water.
14. Whenever possible, buy and eat organically raised foods.
15. To lose weight, reduce both carbohydrates and calories.

—⟋⟋⟍—

The Anti-Inflammation Syndrome Step 1: Eat a Variety of Fresh and Whole Foods

Most of the following steps are more specific versions of this first one: eat a variety of fresh and whole foods. These are foods that are in or close to their original state. They have not been processed or altered beyond refrigeration, kitchen preparation, and cooking. In other words such foods look pretty much the way they did in nature (which is not how processed foods look). A couple of examples should help clarify the meaning of fresh and whole foods.

A freshly broiled piece of fish *looks, smells,* and *tastes* like a piece of fish. It is very different from breaded and deep-fried fish, which is coated in refined flour and then cooked in a mix of vegetable and partially hydrogenated vegetable oils.

A piece of baked chicken still looks like a part of a chicken, which breaded and deep-fried chicken nuggets do not.

A carrot looks like a carrot, which carrot juice (devoid of fiber) does not.

An apple looks like an apple, which applesauce and apple juice do not.

A baked potato looks like a potato, which French fries (boiled in hydrogenated or oxidized oils) do not.

In practice, avoid any food that does not resemble what it looked like as it was growing or being raised. (The exceptions are foods that have just been cut up or prepared in a food processor or blender.) Following this principle means that you will have to strictly limit foods sold in boxes, cans, jars, and bottles—often, even those sold in health and natural-food stores. The reason is that boxing, canning, and bottling usually indicate some sort of processing or alteration from the food's original state, plus the addition of unwanted ingredients such as sugars, refined grains, most oils, flavor enhancers, texturizers, and more. Canned vegetables may or may not have added sugar; regardless, they are less nutritious than frozen, and frozen vegetables are usually less nutritious than fresh.

So as you stare into your cupboard, you must be wondering what you will eat. It's simple: fresh (or frozen) fish, lean meats, spices and herbs for seasoning, lots of vegetables, and some fruit. Such foods are straightforward, uncomplicated, and easy to prepare and vary.

The Anti-Inflammation Syndrome Step 2: Eat More Fish, Especially Cold-Water Varieties

Cold-water fish contain the largest amounts of the most biologically active, "preformed" omega-3 fatty acids. Preformed means that the fatty acids exist as eicosapentaenoic acid (EPA) and docosahexaenoic acid (DHA), and the body does not have to make them from alpha-linolenic acid. This shortcut enables your body to put the anti-inflammatory properties of EPA and DHA to work right away.

An ideal amount of dietary omega-3 fatty acids is about 7 grams a week, which you can obtain in two to three servings of fish. Of course, eating fish more often is even better, particularly during the first couple months of the Anti-Inflammation Syndrome Diet Plan. (Fish oil supplements, which will be discussed in chapter 8, also can rapidly boost your intake of EPA and DHA.)

The fish with the highest concentrations of omega-3 fatty acids are mackerel, Pacific herring, anchovy, lake trout, king salmon, and Atlantic salmon. Tuna, halibut, cod, sole, snapper, crab, and shrimp contain smaller quantities of omega-3 fatty acids, but they are still healthy. Wild salmon contains a higher portion of anti-inflammatory omega-3 fatty acids compared with farmed salmon. All types of Alaskan salmon—including king, coho, and sokeye—are always wild. By 2004, labeling laws will require distributors to identify whether the salmon was wild or farmed.

Although fresh fish is always better (and smells less fishy) than frozen, most fish is delivered frozen to supermarkets. You may be broil, bake, poach, grill, or pan fry the fish in olive oil (and you should specify one of these when ordering in restaurants). Never eat breaded and deep-fried fish. The breading adds empty calories, and the frying saturates the breading and fish with highly processed, pro-inflammatory omega-6 and trans fatty acids. At home, you can also stir fry a dense fish in olive oil.

If you do not like the taste of fish (or are a vegetarian), you can increase your intake of EPA and DHA in other ways. Freshly ground flaxseed sprinkled on a salad or vegetables, or flaxseed oil drizzled on them, contains large amounts of alpha-linolenic acid. Of course, your body will have to convert it to EPA and DHA. In addition, you can eat eggs enriched with omega-3 fatty acids or one of the growing number of products containing deodorized fish oils, such as some types of Millina's Finest tomato sauces.

The Issue of Mercury in Fish

Some types of fish absorb mercury, a toxic metal. So how do you address this issue when eating anti-inflammatory fish?

One way is to avoid fish that you know are from polluted waters. Farm-raised fish are likely free of mercury, though they have the disadvantage of having slightly more omega-6 fatty acids compared with wild fish (because farm-raised fish are fed grains). A second way to deal with this problem is to take selenium supplements. Garry F. Gordon, M.D., of Payson, Arizona, an expert on heavy metal toxicity, points out that selenium binds with mercury and blocks its toxicity.

Taking selenium supplements might not be a bad idea in general, because this essential mineral boosts antioxidant levels in the body, which will have an anti-inflammatory effect. A daily supplement containing 200 mcg of selenium supplements (preferably the high-selenium yeast form, which will be identified on the label) makes good sense.

Mercury, however, is not an issue with fish-oil supplements. A ConsumerLab.com analysis of different brands of fish-oil capsules found no detectable amounts of mercury.

The Anti-Inflammation Syndrome Step 3: Eat Meat from Free-Range or Grass-Fed Animals

The animals that provided meat to Paleolithic peoples ate grass and leaves, which are rich sources of alpha-linolenic acid. For this reason, game meat contains large amounts of anti-inflammatory omega-3 fatty acids. Today, when farm animals are fed corn and other grains, their muscles contain almost no omega-3 fatty acids and substantial amounts of saturated fats.

It is important to avoid, or strictly limit your intake of, meat from corn-fed animals. This caution often applies to meat or eggs from "vegetarian-fed" animals, which may be corn-fed. Many natural foods stores, such as the Wild Oats and Whole Foods chains, have full-service meat departments, and many of their meats are from grass-fed or free-range animals. Similarly, chicken, turkey, and duck should come from animals that were allowed to peck around for their natural diet, not fed corn and other grains. Always ask your butcher to be sure. See appendix B for sources of meat from grass-fed animals.

The Anti-Inflammation Syndrome Step 4: Eat a Lot of Vegetables, the More Colorful the Better

Vegetables and many fruits are the best dietary sources of antioxidants, which help dampen overactive immune responses. Contrary to popular opinion, most of these antioxidants are not vitamins. The lion's share are a large family of vitaminlike nutrients known as polphenolic flavonoids.

More than five thousand flavonoids (one subfamily among polyphenols) have been identified in plants. Quercetin, one particular anti-inflammatory flavonoid, is found in apples and onions. A small apple (about 3.5 oz) contains approximately 5.7 mg of vitamin C, but more than 500 mg of antioxidant polyphenols and flavonoids, which together are equivalent to 1,500 mg of vitamin C.

In addition, vegetables and fruit are also rich sources of carotenoids, another class of powerful antioxidants. Although more than six hundred carotenoids have been found in nature, only a handful appear important for humans. These include alpha-carotene, beta-carotene, lutein, and lycopene.

The rule to follow is diversity. Eat at least five servings of vegetables or fruit daily, and make a point of eating different types. Try to eat one large salad daily, made with dark leafy green lettuces (not iceberg lettuce, which was created in 1903 to withstand damage in shipping) or spinach, tomatoes, scallions, shredded carrots, and other vegetables. You can certainly add some grilled chicken, fish, or shrimp to the salad.

With another meal, steam, sauté, or grill vegetables as a side dish to fish or meat. On one day, you might want to steam broccoli and cauliflower. On another, you can pan fry baby asparagus and green beans in olive oil and garlic. To keep things interesting, on still another day, you might grill or broil slices of squash, eggplant, and fennel, brushing them with olive oil and garlic powder. A little garlic, olive oil, and lemon will enhance the flavor of almost any vegetable.

The Anti-Inflammation Syndrome Step 5:
Use Spices and Herbs to Flavor Foods

For many people salt (sodium chloride) and black pepper are the usual flavor enhancers sprinkled onto foods. The Paleolithic diet contained large amounts of potassium and small amounts of naturally occurring sodium. With large amounts of salt added during the manufacture of food products (once again, carefully read package labels) and still more at the table, today's diets typically contain far more sodium than potassium. Excess intake of sodium can raise blood pressure and interfere with the body's use of calcium.

A variety of spices and herbs adds a palette of flavors to foods. But the benefits of basil, oregano, garlic, and other spices and herbs go beyond taste. Culinary herbs are rich in antioxidant flavonoids and natural Cox-2 inhibitors. While the amounts of spices and herbs in a single meal may not have a substantial anti-inflammatory effect, they enhance an anti-inflammatory dietary regimen.

If you enjoy a pungent kick with some of your foods, substitute a little cayenne powder for black pepper (unless you are allergic to night-shades—see step 8). Cayenne contains substances that block the transmission of pain between nerve cells.

The Anti-Inflammation Syndrome Step 6:
Use Olive Oil as Your Primary Cooking Oil

Extra-virgin olive oil should be your main cooking oil. It is rich in anti-inflammatory oleic acid (an omega-9 fatty acid), vitamin E, and polyphenolic flavonoids. Different brands of olive oil, and olive oil derived from different types of olives, have different flavors, so it is good to try different ones. Always use extra-virgin olive oil, an indicator of high quality, and look for a date on the bottle. The olive oil is best used within a year of picking and bottling, but it can be used for cooking for two to three years.

Although olive oil is a pressed oil, which was not consumed during our Paleolithic development, it is an acceptable compromise for our modern times. The omega-9 fatty acids in olive oil help offset years of excessive omega-6 intake. Olive oil, like fish oil, is also valuable for its potent anti-inflammatory properties. Consider it a "supplement" with an exceptional flavor.

As an alternative to olive oil if you want a cooking oil with a different taste, cold pressed macadamia nut oil is a good substitute. Macadamia nut oil is rich in anti-inflammatory oleic acid, the same omega-9 fat found in olive oil. Australian Mac Nut oil is an excellent product. (See appendix B.) It has a high smoke point, so you can cook with it at higher temperatures than you could with olive oil.

Several other oils or fats in small amounts can be used as well. A little butter adds a nice flavor to many meals, and its saturated fat should not pose a problem as long as you are consuming large amounts of omega-3 fatty acids. Grapeseed oil and canola oil also contain omega-9 and omega-3 fatty acids, and they withstand high cooking temperatures very well. However, most grapeseed and canola oils are obtained through chemical extraction (in contrast to mechanical pressing), which may leave trace amounts of solvents in the oils. Look more carefully in grocery stores and you will likely find mechanically pressed grapeseed and canola oils—although olive oil is still preferable to them.

Do not heat flaxseed or fish oils, and do not use them to cook foods. High temperatures rapidly oxidize and break them down, leading to the formation of pro-inflammatory free radicals. It is all right, of course, to cook fish because its mass resists those high temperatures unless, of course, you happen to overcook or burn it.

The Anti-Inflammation Syndrome Step 7: Avoid Conventional Cooking Oils

Conventional cooking oils, such as corn, peanut, safflower, soybean, sunflower, and cottonseed oils, are high in pro-inflammatory omega-6 fatty acids and contain virtually no anti-inflammatory omega-3 or omega-9 fatty acids. These oils are commonly used in an enormous number of processed and packaged foods, including microwave meals, breakfast bars, salad dressings, and in many restaurants. The extensive use of these cooking oils is largely why the modern diet contains twenty to thirty times more pro-inflammatory than anti-inflammatory oils.

The worst oils are partially hydrogenated vegetable oils. All partially hydrogenated oils contain trans fatty acids, which are considerably more dangerous than saturated fats. Vegetable shortenings and hard margarines are among the worst of such products, but you will find partially hydrogenated oils in salad dressings, nondairy creamers, bakery products, and many processed foods.

It is always wise to carefully read the label of a food package. You are most likely to run into all of these pro-inflammatory oils in fast-food restaurants (McDonald's, Burger King, KFC), Chinese restaurants, and "low end" chain restaurants (Denny's and Carrow's), which rely heavily on processed, ready-to-heat foods.

—⁓—

Navigating Restaurant Food

If you are hoping to follow the Anti-Inflammation Syndrome Diet Plan while eating at fast-food restaurants, the advice is simple: forget it. All of these chains rely on mass-produced food products, which are highly processed and loaded with pro-inflammatory nutrients, such as omega-6 fatty acids, trans fatty acids, sugars, and refined grains.

Family-run ethnic and upscale nouvelle cuisine restaurants often use fresh ingredients, more anti-inflammatory nutrients, and are generally more accommodating when diners ask for modifications to meals. For example, restaurants will usually serve, when asked, a sandwich without bread and substitute some sort of steamed vegetable or a salad for French fries.

Your best bets when eating out are Greek, Italian, and Middle Eastern restaurants. These cuisines typically use olive oil and tasty spices. Most meat and vegetable dishes are safe on the Anti-Inflammation Syndrome Diet Plan, but watch out for the occasional breaded meat or vegetable, as well as for pita bread, falafel, or couscous.

Japanese food also is a good choice, as long as you stick with simple fish dishes or sushi and sashimi. Teriyaki sauces usually contain some sugar, and tempuras are deep fried, though quickly.

Mexican foods tend to include a lot of grains and dairy—common allergens and abundant calories. However, fajitas are generally all right if you avoid the tortillas. Chinese foods are typically stir fried in soybean oil, which is high in pro-inflammatory fats.

—⁓—

The Anti-Inflammation Syndrome Step 8: Identify and Avoid Food Allergens

Food allergies or allergylike food sensitivities can rev up the immune system and contribute to chronic inflammation. It is relatively easy and inexpensive to obtain a "food allergy panel" using a simple blood test. Indeed, the health mobiles that occasionally visit supermarkets can perform allergy panel tests for about $30.

It may be easier to assess your likelihood of being allergic to certain foods when you don't already have an obvious reaction after eating a particular food. The reason is that people often become allergic to the foods they eat most often, for biochemical reasons too involved to discuss here. In addition, food allergies often take the form of a food addiction—such as a food you crave or cannot imagine living without. If you avoid a suspect food and all related foods (such as all foods with dairy) for a week, and you are in fact allergic to it, you will feel better. However, you also might not notice any difference in how you feel until you add that food back to your diet, when you suddenly feel worse.

In *Going Against the Grain,* nutritionist Melissa Diane Smith writes that as many as half of Americans have some degree of gluten intolerance. The gut damage from gluten can predispose people to numerous other food allergies. A damaged, or leaky, gut can allow undigested food proteins to enter the bloodstream, where they trigger an immune response. The most common sources of gluten are wheat, rye, barley, and oats.

Nightshades are another problematic group of foods for many people with rheumatoid arthritis. These foods include tomatoes, potatoes, eggplants, and peppers. Although tobacco is not a food, it is a member of the nightshade family. Before Columbus discovered Native Americans eating tomatoes and peppers, Europeans considered nightshades to be poisonous. Nightshades do contain a variety of mildly toxic compounds and, by some estimates, one of every five arthritics has allergiclike sensitivities to nightshades. Given the prevalence of tomatoes and potatoes (such as ketchup on fries), as well as their inclusion in many processed foods, it is advisable for arthritics to stop eating these foods for several weeks to see if symptoms lessen.

The Anti-Inflammation Syndrome Step 9: Avoid or Strictly Limit Sugars

Refined sugars are the ultimate in empty calories. They provide carbohydrates and calories but no vitamins, minerals, or protein. And sugars appear on labels by a variety of names: sucrose, high-fructose corn syrup, dextrose, glucose, and other names, which reflect slightly different chemical structures or food sources. Even boxes of salt contain a little sugar, and many popular sugar substitutes (NutraSweet, Equal) contain some sugar in the form of maltodextrose.

With two-thirds of all Americans now overweight, there is no justification for people to consume such empty calories. High-sugar and highly refined carbohydrate diets in general elevate levels of pro-inflammatory C-reactive protein (CRP), even in thin people.

For an occasional sweetener, a small amount of honey might suffice; it is far too sweet to consume excessively. Stevia, a noncaloric herbal sweetener available at health food stores, is three hundred times sweeter than sugar and is an excellent sugar substitute. "Raw sugar" is merely dirty white sugar; it contains almost undetectable amounts of a few minerals (which can be better obtained in other, more nutritious foods).

Soft drinks may be the worst single source of sugar and high-fructose corn syrup (a blend of two sugars, sucrose and fructose). Fifty years ago, most soft drinks were sold in tiny 6-ounce bottles. Today, 1-liter cups and 2-liter bottles are common. A 2-liter bottle of Coca-Cola contains almost 0.5 cup of sugars in the form of high-fructose corn syrup. Even worse, a 2-liter bottle of Sunkist orange soda contains considerably more than 0.5 cup of sugars. The Center for Science in the Public Interest, a consumer organization, has accurately described soft drinks as "liquid candy." The *average* American consumes 53 gallons of soft drinks a year, and a total of about 150 pounds of refined sugars, thus heavily contributing to this pro-inflammatory profile. Because these amounts are averages, many people consume far greater amounts of soft drinks and sugars.

The Anti-Inflammation Syndrome Step 10: Avoid or Limit Refined Grains

Like sugars, refined grains provide mostly empty calories, even though many grain products have been "enriched" with a few vitamins. The most common grain in the Western diet is wheat, used to make bread, pasta, muffins, bagels, cookies, and a near-infinite variety of pastries. Many processed foods contain a combination of refined grains, sugars, and partially hydrogenated vegetable oils.

Some people might argue that whole-wheat bread is far superior to refined white bread. While whole-wheat bread does contain more fiber and a few more vitamins and minerals, it also contains more antinutrients, such as lectins. Lectins, a family of proteins, interfere with the absorption of vitamins and minerals and, in some people, stimulate unneeded immune cell activity. According to Loren Cordain, Ph.D., of Colorado State University at Fort Collins and author of *The Paleo Diet,* lectins may exacerbate the abnormal immune response at the heart of rheumatoid arthritis.

Overall, grains are a poor substitute for the greater nutritional value of vegetables.

White rice is similar to refined white bread in that most of its important nutrients have been refined out and mostly carbohydrate is left. Brown rice is far superior, although it, too, contains some lectins. Although relatively high in carbohydrate, it also contains vitamins, minerals, protein, and fiber, and no gluten.

It is not necessary to eliminate all grains when on the Anti-Inflammation Syndrome Diet Plan, unless you are sensitive to gluten. However, it is wise to greatly reduce their intake so they are only an occasional treat. If nothing else, large quantities of grains, such as in the form of breads and pastas, displace far more nutritious foods.

—m—

Navigating the Supermarket

In *Syndrome X: The Complete Nutritional Program to Prevent and Reverse Insulin Resistance,* my coauthors and I provided detailed instructions for shopping at supermarkets and natural foods markets. The best way to navigate supermarkets is simple: shop along the perimeter.

Nearly all supermarkets follow a similar floor plan, with refrigerated foods (produce, meat, and dairy) on the perimeter, and heavily processed foods in the center of the store. Fresh foods generally require refrigeration, and you will want to do most of your food shopping in the produce, meat, and fish departments.

As you move toward the center of the store, you will find entire aisles dedicated to soft drinks, cookies, breads, and cereals. All of these foods are incompatible with the Anti-Inflammation Syndrome Diet Plan. The same is true for the frozen-food aisles, typically located right in the middle. The freezers usually are filled with variations of ice cream, high-sugar juices, and highly processed microwave meals.

—m—

The Anti-Inflammation Syndrome Step 11: Limit Your Intake of Dairy Products

Dairy products, with the exception of mother's milk during infancy, is another recent addition to the human diet. Many people, particularly Asians and Africans, lose the ability to digest milk after childhood. In addition, no species on Earth naturally consumes the milk of another species, with the exception of people. In terms of chemical composition, cow's milk is intended to nurture calves, not humans of any age.

Cow's milk also is a common allergen. It provides considerable saturated fat, and some people have argued that homogenization alters the size and metabolism of milk fat, making it more likely to promote heart disease. As beverages, milk and milk shakes provide a large quantity of calories, when the body really requires only water.

Small amounts of cheeses may be all right for many people, unless they are allergic to dairy. Cheeses do provide concentrated protein, but most of their fat is saturated because cows are fed grains rather than simply allowed to feed on grass. However, given the evolutionary implications of dairy consumption, it is best to limit your intake of milk and other dairy products.

The Anti-Inflammation Syndrome Step 12: Snack on Nuts and Seeds

So what do you do with your sweet tooth? Try eating more nuts, such as almonds, cashews, filberts, macadamias, and pistachios, as well as seeds, such as pumpkin seeds. Nuts and seeds are relatively high in fat, a mix of both linoleic and alpha-linolenic acids, and their fat content provides a sweet taste. In particular, almond butter tastes very sweet and is less allergenic than peanuts (although people sensitive to peanuts must make sure that there is no trace of peanuts in almond butter).

Studies have found that regularly eating nuts (preferably raw or dry roasted) reduces the risk of heart disease. One reason for this may be that nuts are very filling and can displace foods with saturated fat. Also, nuts and seeds are also rich in many minerals such as magnesium that are necessary for a healthy heart.

The Anti-Inflammation Syndrome Step 13: When Thirsty, Drink Water

Water is the beverage virtually all animals—again, except for people—consume for life. If you live in an urban area and the quality or taste of tap water leaves a lot to be desired, drink filtered water. Both the Brita and Pur systems filter out chlorine, heavy metals, and, unfortunately, even some of the dietary minerals (such as calcium and magnesium). Buy a brand of sparkling mineral water with a particularly high mineral content, such as Gerolsteiner. Scientists have found that drinking high-mineral water immediately triggers a series of bone-building biochemical reactions. A wedge of lime or lemon adds a citrus flavor to the water, whether sparkling or still.

While water should be your main drink, another beverage option is tea. Various teas—black, green, and herbal—provide antioxidant polyphenol flavonoids, which have been shown to reduce the risk of heart disease and cancer. Some research has also found that the topical application of green tea (cooled down, of course) can reverse some types of dermatitis. It is easy to make iced tea simply by refrigerating warm tea or sun tea.

And what of coffee, the beverage consumed each day by the majority of Westerners? Although the research is contradictory, the risk of health problems does seem to increase when more than a couple of cups of coffee are consumed daily. Some research indicates that the caffeine in coffee and many teas may stimulate inflammation, so it might be worthwhile eliminating caffeinated beverages for a week or two and seeing how you feel.

Some research has shown that red wines, because of their high antioxidant content, may reduce the risk of coronary artery disease. Other alcoholic beverages, such as spirits, have a deleterious effect on health, largely because they are liver toxins and provide no nutritional value. Moderate amounts of red wine, such as a couple of glasses per week, should be fine on the Anti-Inflammation Syndrome Diet Plan.

The best guidance is to drink mostly water and a little tea. And, as noted in step 9, avoid all soft drinks and other beverages (including energy drinks and so-called quick thirst quenchers) that contain sugar, high-fructose corn syrup, or other caloric sweeteners.

—⁂—

Smoking and Inflammation

Virtually everyone who smokes (or chews) tobacco products knows that they are hazardous to health. In addition to increasing the risk of lung cancer, tobacco smoke boosts the risk of many other types of cancer, emphysema, and coronary artery disease. Smoking significantly elevates levels of C-reactive protein (CRP), a powerful promoter of inflammation. Even after a person stops smoking, his or her CRP levels remain higher than normal for years. If you don't smoke, don't start. And if you do, try to break the habit.

—⁂—

The Anti-Inflammation Syndrome Step 14: Buy and Eat Organically Raised Foods

Organic foods are produced without any synthetic pesticides in an environmentally sustainable fashion. That means, essentially, that the soil quality is preserved and enhanced, which is in sharp contrast to conventional farming practices. Organic foods are generally a little more expensive than conventional foods. Consider organics as a desirable option when you can afford them.

There are two justifications for considering organics. One is that they are free of pesticides and genetically engineered material. Many pesticides are estrogen mimics, meaning that they simulate the effect of estrogen and may disrupt the actions of our own hormones. Although pesticides may or may not influence inflammation, it may be best to act conservatively and avoid exposure to them.

The second justification is that several small research studies have found that organic vegetables and fruit tend to have higher vitamin and mineral levels, compared with conventional produce. And, although this is a subjective judgment, many people feel that organics taste better than conventional vegetables and fruit.

Finally, if you eat meat from free-range or grass-fed animals, it is likely to be free of pesticides. Often, corn and other grains intended for farm animals are not organic, and they are also treated with pesticides to prevent destruction by insects. So, for many reasons, it is best to opt for organic foods when obtainable and affordable.

The Anti-Inflammation Syndrome Step 15: To Lose Weight, Reduce Both Carbohydrates and Calories

Sixty-five percent—two-thirds—of Americans are now overweight. In addition, 31 percent—more than one-fourth—of Americans also are obese, that is, more than thirty pounds over their ideal weight. In 2002 scientists reported that overweight is increasing worldwide, largely the result of Americans exporting their unhealthy food habits to other nations.

Fat cells, particularly the type that form around the abdomen, produce large amounts of two powerful inflammation-causing substances, interleukin-6 and C-reactive protein. These high levels of inflammatory compounds are a big part of the reason why being overweight greatly increases a person's risk of diabetes, heart disease, osteoarthritis, and other inflammatory disorders.

Eating according to the Anti-Inflammation Syndrome Diet Plan will likely lead to some weight loss. This is because the diet discourages the use of convenience and fast foods, which contain large amounts of calories and carbohydrates relative to protein, vitamins, minerals, good fats, and fiber. Another reason is that calories from anti-inflammatory omega-3 and omega-9 fatty acids are not converted to body fat as readily as calories from omega-6 fatty acids and saturated fats.

Still, you may wish to further reduce your weight on the Anti-Inflammation Syndrome Diet Plan. You can accomplish this by modifying the diet plan so it is a little more consistent with the weight-loss recommendations in my previous book *Syndrome X: The Complete Nutritional Program to Prevent and Reverse Insulin Resistance.* Some compelling research suggests that the worst possible diet (in terms of Syndrome X, diabetes, and weight gain) is one high in both refined carbohydrates and saturated fats—that is, the typical American diet. So the reasonable alternative is an anti-inflammatory diet that further restricts carbohydrates and saturated fats.

To put these ideas into practice and to lose weight, you will need to eliminate all or nearly all grain-based foods, including whole grains, since these foods (as well as foods with refined sugars) are the principal source of dietary calories and carbohydrates. (This is easier than you might think. I lost twenty pounds and four inches from my waist after giving up pasta.) In addition, you might curtail your intake of legumes, because they also contain substantial amounts of carbohydrates.

Although these recommendations have similarities to the Atkins diet, they are very different. It is important to replace these grain- and legume-based carbohydrates with ample quantities of nonstarchy or low-starch vegetables and fruit. Such foods include spinach, broccoli, cauliflower, lettuces, tomatoes, cucumbers, apples, and berries. Basically, one large salad daily (with an olive oil dressing) and sides of vegetables or fruit with lunch and dinner should provide modest amounts of carbohydrates and respectable quantities of fiber. To lower your intake of saturated fat, eat less beef, pork, and lamb, but increase your consumption of fish, chicken, and turkey.

Physical activity is important as well. Numerous studies have found that going for a walk each day improves insulin function and lowers blood sugar levels, which also contribute to maintaining normal weight. Going for a thirty-minute walk each day is sufficient, though longer walks and more vigorous exercise will yield greater benefits. If you engage in regular exercise, bear in mind that muscle weighs more than fat.

Therefore, you may gain a little weight, even though you are trimmer or more muscular.

If you happen to lose more weight than you wish, you can increase your intake of nutritious unrefined carbohydrates, such as those in brown rice, sweet potatoes, yams, and squash. As with any diet, you will have to make individual adjustments. Your guideposts are how you feel and how you look.

The following pyramid illustrates the points made in this chapter.

The Anti-Inflammation Syndrome Food Pyramid

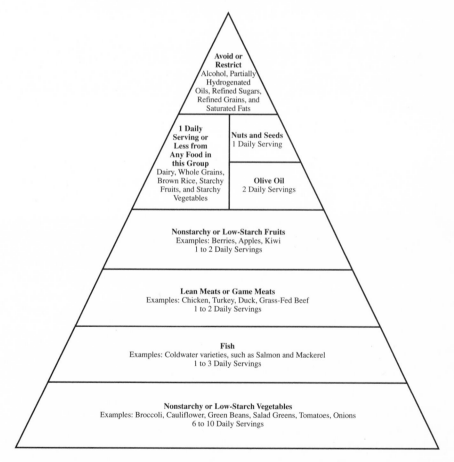

Because of the widespread use of the U.S. Department of Agriculture's food pyramid, this drawing might help some people visualize the Anti-Inflammation Syndrome Food Pyramid. Foods toward the top are those you would eat the least of, whereas those toward the bottom are those you would eat the most of.

CHAPTER 7

Anti-Inflammation Syndrome Menu Plans and Recipes

By following most or all of the anti-inflammation dietary steps, you will find that it is relatively easy to order healthy meals in many restaurants. However, you may be wondering about what to cook at home. This chapter offers a number of recipes for breakfast, lunch, and dinner, as well as a sample seven-day menu plan. This menu plan is merely a guideline and is not meant as a strict rule for what you must eat on any given day. Overall, this chapter takes a very positive approach to food selection, emphasizing what you should eat instead of what you should not.

Unlike many diet plans that are extremely rigid, the Anti-Inflammation Syndrome Diet Plan encourages flexibility and creativity in cooking and food choices. Inflexible dietary regimens can, for many people, become difficult to follow, and such plans often beg to be violated. So, in following the recipes in this chapter, please feel comfortable adjusting quantities, particularly of spices, to suit your personal tastes.

It is worthwhile keeping several guidelines in mind when preparing anti-inflammatory meals at home.

1. You will have to plan some of your major meals generally one to two days in advance. Poor meal planning has become very common and, combined with hunger pangs, often leads to picking the fastest meal

obtainable—a pizza, burger and fries, or microwave lunch or dinner—which are typically rich in pro-inflammatory ingredients. Making a fresh, anti-inflammatory dinner will not take a long time if you have done a modicum of planning. You can do this planning with a pen and pad of paper during television commercials, during a break at work, and perhaps while commuting. You can also stimulate your culinary creativity by thumbing through cookbooks in bookstores.

2. Keep your meals simple if you have time constraints. Many diet books and cookbooks contain extraordinarily complex recipes, with five or ten different spices and intricate preparation. Relatively few of us have the time to prepare such meals, except perhaps on a weekend or for a special occasion. With this situation in mind, the recipes in this chapter contain relatively few ingredients and are easy to prepare. Still, some people may complain that the following recipes—as simple as they are—take too much time. They certainly do take more time than a microwave meal or driving through a fast-food restaurant. But as with everything else in life, you are faced with choices: Do you want to continue living the way that made you sick, or do you want to take the steps needed to be healthy?

3. With the time you invest in making a major meal, such as dinner, it is efficient to scale up (i.e., to double) the quantities so you have great-tasting leftovers. Leftovers have gotten a bad reputation—often deserved—because reheated junk foods often taste much worse than when originally heated. However, leftovers from tasty meals usually remain tasty the second time around. They can be quickly spruced up, reheated, or used in still other recipes—what one friend refers to as "planovers." For example, leftovers from a chicken or turkey dinner can be used in a quick-to-prepare breakfast or a brown-bag lunch at the office. In addition, some recipes, such as the Tomato-Free Ratatouille, are meant as both a side dish with dinner and as part of breakfast.

4. It is worthwhile experimenting and trying to be creative in the kitchen, modifying recipes as you go. Methodically measuring out every single ingredient—3 tablespoons or this and ½ teaspoon of that—may be a good method while learning the basics of cooking, but sometimes being a little less precise can make cooking more *fun*. I say this as a man who did not learn how to cook until age forty-nine. After learning some of the basics and also making some mistakes, I discovered that cooking is enjoyable and creative. If I can do this, you can also, regardless of your circumstances.

As with any creative pursuit, set aside some time, and approach cooking as a personally rewarding activity, not a stressful chore. It helps to envision all of your ingredients—meat or fish, vegetables, condiments, and spices—as comparable to the palette of paints used by an artist. Of course, some foods (like colors) work better together than others. If you are not used to cooking, it may take several months to develop this level of comfort, but along the way you will gain a sense of accomplishment and greater confidence from the tasty meals you create.

5. To stimulate your interest in culinary experiments, read other recipe books for ideas, and watch the Food Network (www.foodtv.com) on television to learn new cooking techniques and recipes. It is relatively easy to experiment and modify many conventional recipes to the principles of the Anti-Inflammation Syndrome Diet Plan. For example, you can substitute olive oil for nearly any other cooking oil, and often you can use rice flour instead of wheat flour for dredging chicken and fish.

6. Many of the dinner recipes emphasize fish because of their rich reservoir of anti-inflammatory compounds. If you hate the taste of fish, don't give up. Follow the other dietary principles and be sure to take fish oil capsules to obtain the necessary eicosapentaenoic acid (EPA) and docosahexaenoic acid (DHA). You might also try just one fish recipe, such as fresh tuna, to determine whether you genuinely dislike fish or whether you have simply had bad experiences with fish. Fresh fish does not have a strong fishy odor.

Anti-Inflammation Syndrome Diet Plan Meals

The recipes are organized counterintuitively, with dinner first, followed by dinner side dishes, and then by lunch and breakfast. There is a reason for this type of flow. Dinner leftovers, used creatively, can be used in making lunches and breakfasts, thus saving considerable time preparing other meals. All of these recipes can be easily doubled, so you have plenty of tasty leftovers.

—⁂—

Quick Tip: Natural Flavor Enhancers

To enhance the flavor of almost any fish or fowl, add some olive oil, garlic, or fresh-squeezed lemon juice. Oregano and basil also add a lot of flavor, as long as they do not compete with other spices and herbs (such as herbes de Provence or dill).

—⁂—

Dinner Main Courses

Baked Salmon *(Serves 2)*

> olive oil
> 2 salmon fillets, about 4 to 6 ounces each
> basil, to taste
> oregano, to taste
> 1 to 3 teaspoons basalmic vinaigrette, to taste

Preheat the oven to 350 degrees.

Coat the bottom of a baking dish with olive oil. Rinse and pat excess water off the salmon, and place them in the baking dish. Apply a thin coat of olive oil on top of the fillets (to add flavor and to prevent burning). Sprinkle basil and oregano to taste on the fillets. Drizzle the balsamic vinaigrette on the fillets. Bake for approximately 10 minutes. The cooking time may vary by a couple of minutes, depending on the oven and thickness of the fillets, so examine after 8 minutes to ensure that they are not burning or undercooked. The baked salmon goes well with Spinach and Leek Sauté (page 89) and Flavorful Brown Rice (page 89).

Pumpkin Seed Crusted Halibut *(Serves 2)*

> ½ teaspoon coriander
> ¼ cup raw pumpkin seeds, chopped
> ¼ cup olive oil
> 1 pound halibut, cut into two pieces
> 2 pats butter
> 1 lemon
> 1 tablespoon parsley

Preheat the oven to 350 degrees.

Add the coriander to the pumpkin seeds, then chop the seeds in a food processor, being careful to avoid a flourlike texture. Meanwhile, spread the olive oil over the bottom of baking dish. Dredge the halibut through the olive oil so all sides of the fish are lightly coated. With one hand, spoon the chopped pumpkin seeds onto all sides of the fish, while using the fingers of your other hand to pat the seeds onto the fish. Add one pat of butter to the top of each piece of fish. Bake the fish 10 minutes per inch of thickness. When done, squeeze lemon juice on each piece of fish, and sprinkle with parsley.

—സ—

Quick Tip: Sanitary Gloves

Preparing food can often get a little messy. To avoid having to repeatedly wash your hands (such as after handling fish or rubbing olive oil into fish or meats), wear disposable, sanitary plastic gloves. Large quantities of these gloves are available inexpensively at Price-Costco and many other stores. Using these gloves also reduces possible bacterial contamination of your hands and the food.

—സ—

Pan Fried Swordfish with Citrus Marinade *(Serves 2)*

2 swordfish steaks, approximately 1 pound total
2 tablespoons olive oil

Marinade
1 tablespoon olive oil
2 scallions, diced
1 large lemon, juiced
1 lime, juiced
½ orange, juiced (optional)
4 cloves garlic
1 teaspoon ground coriander
⅛ teaspoon cumin

Prepare the marinade by mixing the marinade ingredients.

Trim the skin from the swordfish and soak in the marinade, refrigerating for 1 to 2 hours. When ready to cook, drain off as much liquid as possible from the marinade. Heat a frypan on medium heat with olive oil, then add the swordfish, with the remainder of the marinade next to the fish. Cook approximately 3 minutes per side. Serve with vegetables and rice.

Simple Poached Salmon *(Serves 4)*

> 1 quart water
> 1 cup vermouth
> 1 onion, sliced
> 1 carrot, sliced
> 1 stalk celery, sliced
> 1 bay leaf
> 1 teaspoon RealSalt or sea salt
> 1 pinch of ground black pepper
> 1 large fillet of salmon with skin on one side
> 1 lemon

Fill a large, low-profile pot with water. Add the vermouth, onion, carrot, celery, bay leaf, salt, and pepper. Bring to a boil, then simmer for 20 minutes. Meanwhile, completely wrap the salmon in a strip of cheesecloth. Fold the cheesecloth so you can unwrap it slightly to check the fish, and leave the ends long enough to drape over the sides of the pan.

Insert the fish into the simmering broth, ideally with 1 inch or 2 inches of water above it. Be careful to keep the ends of the cheesecloth away from the flame or heating element. Bring the water to a boil again, then simmer. Allow 8 minutes per pound for the fish to cook. Unwrap the fish to test with a fork whether it is flaky and done. If it is not done, simmer for a couple more minutes and check again.

When the fish is cooked, lift it out of the pot by grabbing it with the two ends of the cheesecloth. Place the fish on a platter and remove the cheesecloth. Squeeze lemon juice on fish for additional flavor. The fish can be eaten with a Greek-style Tzatziki cucumber-yogurt sauce (available at many supermarkets or ethnic grocers) or a mayonnaise-based sauce (find one at a natural foods grocer), along with vegetables and rice.

Baked Shrimp and Scallops *(Serves 2)*

> olive oil
> 4 to 6 garlic cloves, diced

2 scallions, diced
12 large shrimp, peeled and cleaned
8 large scallops, sliced in half
1 teaspoon each Deliciously Dill spice mix (sold under The Spice
   Hunter label) or oregano and basil
1 lemon, juiced

Coat a large nonstick frypan or wok with olive oil. Sauté garlic and scallions. When the scallions soften, add the shrimp, scallops, and spices. (The scallops should be sliced in half so they cook at the same rate as the shrimp.) Add lemon juice to create a flavorful sauce. The shrimp are cooked when they turn pink on all sides. Serve with rice and vegetables, or toss with a baked spaghetti squash.

Wonderful Baked Chicken Breasts *(Serves 2)*

1 whole or 2 half chicken breasts, boneless
   and skinless
1 cup chicken broth
½ cup olive oil
1 lemon
3 large or 6 small garlic cloves, diced
1 shallot, diced
1 heaping tablespoon of capers
2 tablespoons dried oregano
1 tablespoon dried basil

Preheat oven to 350 degrees.

Trim excess fat and gristle from the chicken. It's all right if the chicken pieces vary in size. If the breasts are thick, carefully slice them laterally, so they end up about half as thick (about ¼ inch each). Spread out the chicken slices and pieces in a baking pan. Next, add the chicken broth, then drizzle the olive oil over the chicken. Cut the lemon, and squeeze the juice over the chicken. Add the garlic, shallots, capers, oregano, and basil. Bake for 30 to 35 minutes. This is an easy-to-prepare and very flavorful dinner and can be served with Pan Fried Veggies (page 90) and Flavorful Brown Rice (page 89).

—⁓—

Quick Tip: Using a Natural Salt

It is important for many people to reduce their intake of salt (sodium chloride). Unfortunately, most salt is added to foods during their manufacture, long before they reach the dining table. In Paleolithic times people consumed far more potassium than sodium, but today people tend to consume far more sodium than potassium. The biggest step in reducing your salt intake is to avoid processed and prepackaged foods, convenience foods, and fast foods. Unprocessed foods—fish, fowl, and vegetables—generally provide more potassium than sodium.

Still, if you would like to use a little salt—just a little—with your meals, try RealSalt. This product, which is extracted from an ancient seabed in southern Utah, contains trace amounts of many minerals. It is available at nearly all health and natural food stores. For more information go to www.realsalt.com.

—⁓—

Evan's Chicken Schnitzel *(Serves 2–3)*

This meal is similar to a chicken fried steak. However, instead of using wheat flour or bread crumbs, you should use Lotus Foods' Bhutanese Red Rice Flour, or order it directly from www.lotusfoods.com. The rice flour is much lighter than wheat; browns nicely; and adds a wonderful, rich flavor.

    1 to 1½ pounds chicken breasts, boneless and skinless
    1 egg, beaten in a bowl
    ¼ cup Bhutanese Red Rice Flour (potato flour can be substituted)
    olive oil
    pat of butter (optional)

Trim excess fat and gristle from the chicken. Slice into thin pieces, running the length of each chicken breast so the pieces are no more than about ¼ inch thick. Dip each piece into the egg, then dredge through the flour. When all of the chicken pieces are prepared (you can prepare very small pieces of chicken similarly to minimize waste), heat the olive oil (and butter, if you choose) in a nonstick frypan. Place the chicken in the pan, cooking about 2 minutes or less per side. Serve with rice and your choice of vegetables.

Saffron Chicken Stir-Fry *(Serves 2–3)*

¼ to ½ teaspoon saffron, ground
¼ cup water
olive oil
pat of butter (optional)
1 to 1½ pounds chicken breast meat, skinless and boneless
6 cloves garlic, diced
1 to 1½ lemons, juiced

To grind the saffron: grind the strands between your fingers in a small bowl. Adding a pinch of salt will help you grind the saffron into a powder. Add water (room temperature or warm) to the bowl with the saffron. Set aside.

Slice or cube the chicken, removing unwanted fat and gristle. Coat a nonstick wok with olive oil (and butter if you wish) over medium heat. Add the chicken and begin stir-frying. When the chicken turns white, add the garlic and saffron mixture and continue to stir-fry for a couple more minutes. Add the lemon juice and stir-fry for another 1 or 2 minutes. The saffron mixture and lemon juice will prevent the chicken from drying out. Serve with rice and vegetables.

Spaghetti Squash Toss *(Serves 1–2)*

This makes for a nice dinner for one or two people, plus leftovers that can be reheated in the microwave for lunch the next day.

1 medium-size spaghetti squash (2 to 2 ½ pounds)
1 boneless, skinless chicken breast or 10 to 20 shrimp and scallops
olive oil
4 to 6 garlic cloves, diced
1 teaspoon basil
1 teaspoon oregano

2 to 3 ounces fresh baby spinach leaves
1 to 2 lemons, juiced
1 lime, juiced
½ orange, juiced
RealSalt (or sea salt) and black pepper, to taste

Bake the spaghetti squash for 1 hour or so, at 350 to 375 degrees, until the skin is soft to the touch. (Use a pot holder or fork to touch it.) Remove the squash from the oven, cut in half lengthwise, and use a spoon to scoop out the seeds. Run a fork along the fruit so you create spaghettilike strands. While the squash is baking, stir-fry the chicken or shrimp and scallops in olive oil along with the garlic, basil, and oregano in a frypan over medium heat. Add the spinach and continue to stir-fry. Add the lemon, lime, and orange juices when the meat is almost cooked. Serve on top of the spaghetti squash. Add RealSalt and black pepper to taste. The stir-frying should take no more than 5 to 10 minutes, so you can time it for when the squash will be ready.

—⁂—

Quick Tip: Quality Chicken Broths

When using packaged chicken broth in a recipe, quality makes a big difference. Health Valley and Pacific organic free-range chicken broths are simple and tasty, without thickeners and excessive amounts of salt. Both brands are available at natural foods grocery stores.

—⁂—

Baked Turkey Breast Provençal *(Serves 4)*

1 turkey breast, on bone or boneless (2 ½ to 3 pounds)
herbes de Provence
rubbed or finely ground dried sage
chicken broth
2 bay leaves
2 tablespoons olive oil, plus additional as needed
1 lemon, juiced
water

Preheat the oven to 350 degrees.

Place the turkey breast in a deep roasting pot, and use your hands to separate but not completely detach the skin from the top of the turkey. Rub a little olive oil on the turkey to keep it from burning or drying out. Sprinkle on herbes de Provence and sage, then place the skin over the spices. You may add a little more olive oil and spices to the skin if you wish. Add about ½ an inch high-quality chicken broth (such as Health Valley or Pacific organic free-range chicken broth) to the bottom of the pot. Add a little more of the spices, plus the bay leaves, 2 tablespoons olive oil, and lemon juice. Bake uncovered for 30 to 40 minutes per pound, approximately 90 minutes to 2 hours total. Add water every 30 minutes or so to maintain the level of the broth, which will become your au jus. During the final 30 minutes, cover the pot. Save leftover turkey and au jus for other meals or recipes, such as Turkey Rice Soup (page 94).

Saffron Seafood Soup *(Serves 4)*

> 1 small onion, finely diced
> 1 leek, very thinly sliced (white part only)
> 1 carrot, thinly sliced
> 2 teaspoons butter
> ½ cup dry vermouth or dry white wine
> 3 to 4 cups fish stock
> 1 cup short-grain brown rice, already cooked
> 0.01 ounce saffron, ground
> ½ teaspoon dried dill or Deliciously Dill seasoning
> ½ to 1 cup heavy cream
> 4 ounces salmon filet, cut into small pieces
> 6 to 8 large shrimp, cut into small pieces
> 1 to 2 oysters, shucked and rinsed
> ½ teaspoon RealSalt or sea salt

Sauté the onion, leek, and carrot in butter in a large saucepan over medium heat. When they soften (3 to 5 minutes), add the vermouth, fish stock, rice, and saffron. Bring to a boil, then add the dill and let simmer for 10 to 15 minutes. (If you prefer to have a thick rather than chunky soup, allow to cool slightly and pureé until smooth, then continue simmering.) Stir the cream into the simmering soup, then add the salmon, shrimp, oysters, and RealSalt. Simmer for another 3 to 5 minutes until the fish is cooked and tender.

Side Dishes

Spinach and Leek Sauté *(Serves 1–2)*

> 1 6-ounce bag fresh spinach
> 1 leek, white part only
> 2 pats of butter
> water
> 1 tablespoon pine nuts
> garlic powder, to taste

Pinch the stems from the spinach leaves and place the leaves in a large colander. Slice the leek into pieces just over the thickness of a quarter. In a 10-inch nonstick frypan, over medium heat, sauté the leek with a pat of butter until the leek starts to caramelize. Meanwhile, boil a pot of water and pour over the spinach in a colander. This will gently wilt and compress the spinach. Allow the spinach to cool a little, then press out the excess water. When the leek starts to caramelize, add the other pat of butter and then the spinach; you may need to use a fork to separate the clumps of spinach. Sauté and add the pine nuts and garlic powder.

This provides a modest vegetable side dish for two people that goes well with Baked Salmon (page 81). Quantities can easily be doubled.

Flavorful Brown Rice *(Serves 2)*

Short-grain brown rice has a wonderful flavor, and at the table you can add a small amount of RealSalt or sea salt and butter to taste.

> 1 cup short-grain brown rice
> 1 cup chicken broth (or plain water)
> 1 cup bottled or filtered water

Rinse the rice in a strainer, then put in a 2-quart saucepan. Add the broth and water (or simply water if you're not using broth). Use very high heat and boil for 5 minutes, then turn the heat down to simmer. The rice should cook fully in about 40 minutes; you may have to adjust the heat above a simmer to accomplish this.

As a variation, consider frying some finely diced shallots, garlic, and onions in as little olive oil as possible, then mixing them into the rice before you start cooking it.

—⁓—

Quick Tip: Nice Rice

Tired of the same old rice? White rice is pretty bland (and nothing more than pure carbohydrate), but brown rice can get a little boring after a while. Lotus Foods (www.lotusfoods.com) markets a selection of rich-tasting rices from Asia that are unlike any other type of rice. The company's Bhutanese Red Rice is a tasty red rice, and Forbidden Rice is a flavorful purple-colored rice. Both types cook faster than brown rice and require less broth (or water), so be careful to follow label directions. Both rices, and others, are also available as flours.

—⁓—

Cauliflower and Broccoli *(Serves 2)*

½ head cauliflower
½ bunch broccoli
½ stick (⅛ pound) butter
2 to 3 tablespoons pine nuts, sliced almonds, or pecan or hazelnut
    pieces

Cut the cauliflower and broccoli into florets about ½ to 1 inch in diameter. Steam in a pot for 10 minutes over high heat. While doing this, melt the butter in a pan, then add nuts of your choice. Transfer the cauliflower and broccoli to a bowl, then pour the butter/nut mixture over and toss. Serve immediately.

Pan Fried Veggies *(Serves 2)*

¼ cup olive oil
1 pat unsalted butter (optional)

1 or 2 small zucchini squashes
1 cup frozen corn kernels
1 large garlic clove, diced
1 scallion, diced
¼ teaspoon garlic powder
½ teaspoon dried oregano
½ teaspoon dried basil
¼ cup pine nuts
1 tablespoon golden raisins

Add olive oil and butter to a 10-inch frypan or wok. Cut the tops and bottoms off the zucchini, quarter them lengthwise, and dice so the pieces are roughly the size of dimes, but a little thicker. Put the zucchini in the pan along with the corn and diced garlic, scallion, garlic powder, oregano, and basil. With a spatula, mix around as you start heating (medium setting) the vegetables. Cover the pan (loosely with a piece of aluminum foil if you don't have a cover). Stir every couple of minutes. After about 5 minutes, add the pine nuts. Cook until the zucchini softens and the corn starts to turn brown and caramelize. After a few minutes more, add the raisins. It should be ready to eat in 10 to 15 minutes. This is an easy side dish and goes great with Wonderful Baked Chicken Breasts (page 84).

—ɯ—

Quick Tip: The Secret of Tomato-Free Ratatouille

Traditional ratatouille consists of sautéed vegetables, including tomatoes. The following recipe avoids tomatoes, a nightshade plant that can aggravate arthritic symptoms in some people. Instead, it uses tomatillos *(Physalis ixocarpa),* also known as Mexican green tomatoes. Tomatillos, which can be bought fresh or canned at supermarkets, are also members of the nightshade family, but they are more closely related to the Cape gooseberry than to tomatoes. If you are very sensitive to nightshades, substitute extra zucchini for the eggplant (another nightshade), and test whether you are sensitive to tomatillos. All of these vegetables cook down, so use a large, covered, nonstick, woklike pan. The amounts below can easily be doubled, allowing the ratatouille to be used as a vegetable side dish and with breakfasts as well. See the Omelette with Tomato-Free

Ratatouille Filling recipe (page 95). Please note: If you react to all night-shade plants, this is not a recipe you should try.

—⚏—

Tomato-Free Ratatouille *(Serves 2–3)*

¼ to ½ cup olive oil
2 small or 1 large eggplant, diced
1 large bell pepper, or the equivalent from several colored
  varieties, diced
2 zucchinis, each about 10 inches long, diced
1 medium red or sweet onion, diced
1 to 2 teaspoons thyme
1 to 2 teaspoons basil
1 bay leaf
4 garlic cloves, finely diced
3 to 4 ripe tomatillos (should have yellow-green lime color), diced
RealSalt or sea salt, to taste

Pour about ¼ cup of olive oil into a pan. Turn the heat to medium. When the olive oil is warm, add the eggplant, stirring occasionally. The eggplant will soak up the olive oil, but keep the pan covered to retain moisture. Add the bell pepper, zucchinis, and onion. After a few minutes, add the thyme, basil, bay leaf, garlic, and tomatillos. Stir occasionally to keep the vegetables from burning, and keep covered when not stirring. Add a little more olive oil if necessary. Turn the heat down and allow to simmer for about 40 minutes or until all of the vegetables are very soft. Add RealSalt or sea salt. Dispose of the bay leaf before serving.

Green Bean and Mushroom Stir-Fry *(Serves 2)*

pat of butter
2 tablespoons olive oil
2 handfuls fresh or frozen green beans, ideally French cut
4 to 5 fresh mushrooms, sliced
garlic powder, to taste
⅛ cup sliced almonds

Heat the butter and olive oil in a nonstick frypan or wok over medium heat. Add the green beans and cook until they start to get soft. Add the mushroom slices and garlic powder. When the green beans and mushrooms are almost cooked, add the sliced almonds.

Mushroom and Spinach Sauté *(Serves 1)*

> olive oil
> 6 to 10 small mushrooms, sliced
> 3 small scallions, diced
> 3 ounces (about ½ bag) fresh spinach
> garlic powder, to taste

Coat a nonstick frypan with olive oil, add the mushrooms and scallions, and sauté over medium heat. Meanwhile, pinch the stems from the spinach leaves (or leave on, if you prefer). When the mushrooms and scallions soften, add the spinach, then add the garlic powder. Stir to thoroughly mix the vegetables together. For variety, use a different type of mushroom, such as shiitake or chanterelle.

Tangy Butternut Squash *(Serves 2)*

> 1 to 2 butternut squashes
> ½ to 1 teaspoon plus additional as needed thyme (dried)
> 1 teaspoon plus additional as needed walnut, hazelnut, or
>   olive oil
> ½ teaspoon balsamic vinegar, plus additional as needed

Preheat oven to 350 degrees.
Cut off the tip of the squash stem, then cut the squash in half lengthwise. Remove the seeds with a spoon (a serrated grapefruit spoon works well). Lightly coat the inside of the squash with olive oil to minimize burning. Place the cut side down (skin side up) on a baking pan, and bake for approximately 1 hour. The squash is cooked when the skin is tender to the touch. (Use a fork or a spoon to touch, not your hand.) Take the squash from the oven, scrape the fruit with a spoon, and place the fruit in a bowl. Add about ½ teaspoon of thyme per squash, plus about 1 teaspoon of walnut or other oil and about ½ teaspoon of basalmic vine-

gar. Mix together with a fork, adding additional thyme, oil, or vinegar to suit your taste.

Lunch Meals

Wonderful Whatever Salad *(Serves 1)*

> any green leafy lettuce (not iceberg) or spinach
> cucumber
> scallion, diced
> tomato or bell peppers
> sliced almonds
> artichoke hearts (packed in water, not oil)
> hemp nut seed
> chicken or turkey diced, or pieces of poached salmon

No amounts are given because they are purely at your discretion. Prepare ingredients in desired amounts and toss. Avoid dressings with soybean oil or hydrogenated vegetable oil. Two recommended salad dressings are Stonewall Kitchen Roasted Garlic Vinaigrette (www.stonewallkitchen. com) and Zeus Greek Salad Dressing (www.zeusfoods.com).

Quick Chicken or Turkey Rice Soup *(Serves 2)*

This soup is a creative, tasty, and adaptable use of leftover chicken or turkey, regardless of how it was originally prepared.

> ⅛ to ¼ cup leftover meat juice
> 2 cups chicken broth
> 2 ounces turkey or chicken
> ½ cup cooked short-grain brown rice
> 1 diced scallion
> ⅓ cup diced mushrooms
> 1 egg, beaten
> garlic powder, to taste
> salt, to taste
> pepper, to taste

Pour meat juice and chicken broth in a saucepan and begin heating. Cut up the chicken or turkey into pieces about ¼ inch in size. Put into the broth along with the rice, scallions, and mushrooms. Stir occasionally and bring to a light boil. Add the egg, which will thicken the soup like an eggdrop soup, and stir occasionally. Cook until the egg starts to turn white. Serve, adding the garlic powder, salt, and pepper at the table.

Breakfasts

Breakfast Scramble *(Serves 1–2)*

> olive oil or butter
> 1 scallion, diced, per person
> spinach (either fresh with stems removed or defrosted)
> 2 tablespoons cooked brown rice
> 1 to 2 tablespoons leftover chicken or turkey, diced
> 2 eggs, beaten, per person

Heat a frypan with olive oil, and sauté the scallions over medium heat until they soften. Add the spinach, brown rice, and pieces of meat. When the spinach is wilted, pour in the eggs and mix thoroughly with a spatula. Serve when the eggs are cooked. Add fresh fruit as a side dish.

Omelette with Tomato-Free Ratatouille Filling *(Serves 1)*

> pat of butter or olive oil
> 2 to 3 eggs
> 2 tablespoons Tomato-Free Ratatouille (page 92)

Heat a pat of butter or a little olive oil in a frypan. Beat and pour the eggs into the pan and begin cooking as a plain omelette. Meanwhile, heat 2 tablespoons of Tomato-Free Ratatouille on a small plate in a microwave. After you flip the omelette, spoon the ratatouille on one side, then fold over the omelette. Serve with fresh fruit, such as berries or apple slices.

Breakfast Mini Chicken Patties *(Serves 2–3)*

1 pound ground chicken (turkey alternative)
4 cloves garlic, diced
4 pitted olives, finely diced
1 tablespoon oregano
1 tablespoon basil

Preheat the oven to 350 degrees.

Put ground chicken in a mixing bowl. (Many natural foods grocers sell ground chicken, frozen, in 1-pound packages.) Add the garlic, olives, oregano, and basil. Mix thoroughly with your hands (wear disposable gloves) and form patties about ¼ inch thick and about the size of an old-fashioned silver dollar (1½ to 2 inches in diameter). One pound of ground chicken should yield about a dozen patties, though you can make them smaller. Place the patties in a baking dish and bake for 20 minutes. When done, soak up extra fat with paper towels.

Tip: Follow the same recipe to make chickenburgers comparable to the size of a hamburger. Use different types of pitted olives (such as green or Kalamata) to vary the flavor. You also can substitute ground turkey for ground chicken.

Breakfast Muesli *(Serves 1)*

This breakfast takes about 5 minutes to prepare the night before and is ready in about 2 minutes in the morning. Use a high-quality muesli, such as the Earth Song Grandpa's Secret Omega-3 Muesli (www. earthsongwholefoods.com). Mix ⅓ cup of muesli with about ½ cup of coconut milk, water, or milk (if you are not allergic to dairy) in a small bowl. Cover the bowl, and leave it in the refrigerator overnight. Meanwhile, defrost a total of 2 to 3 tablespoons of raspberries and blueberries overnight, or be sure to have some fresh fruit on hand for the morning, such as berries, an apple, or a banana. In the morning add the fruit (dice the apple or banana) and mix into the muesli. Add a little cinnamon or a very small amount of nutmeg for flavoring. Eat as a side dish with a few reheated Breakfast Mini Chicken Patties (above).

Baked Sweet Potatoes or Yams *(Serves 1–2)*

    1 to 2 sweet potatoes or yams
    butter
    1 tablespoon fresh chives or scallions, finely diced
    salt, to taste

Preheat the oven to 375 degrees.

Place the potatoes on aluminum foil and bake for 1 to 1½ hours, depending on their size. Cut in half and serve as you would a baked potato, with butter and chives, or scallions. Add salt.

Sample Week-Long Meal Plan

This meal plan is *not* intended as a rigid you-must-follow-or-else dietary plan. Rather, it is just what the name says—a sample of what you might choose to cook, reuse as creative leftovers, or order in a restaurant. The key is following, at every meal, the dietary principles discussed in chapter 6. An asterisk indicates that the recipe is included in this chapter.

Day 1
Breakfast   Breakfast Scramble,* fresh fruit, and a wheat-free waffle with almond butter.

Lunch   In a restaurant, order a grilled chicken breast, minus the bun, and a side of vegetables instead of fries. Sparkling water to drink.

Dinner   Baked Salmon,* Spinach and Leek Sauté,* and rice.

Day 2
Breakfast   Breakfast Mini Chicken Patties,* fresh fruit, and sliced gluten-free bread toasted with almond butter.

Lunch   Wonderful Whatever Salad,* with leftover pieces of salmon from last evening's dinner.

Dinner   Baked Turkey Breast Provençal,* Mushroom and Spinach Sauté,* and rice or baked squash.

Day 3
Breakfast   Leftover Breakfast Mini Chicken Patties,* and Breakfast Musili* with fruit.

Lunch   Reheated turkey with au jus, Spinach and Leek Sauté,* and rice.

Dinner   Pumpkin Seed Crusted Halibut,* Green Bean and Mushroom Stir-Fry,* and Forbidden Rice spinach salad on the side.

Day 4

Breakfast   Omelette with Tomato-Free Ratatouille Filling,* and fresh fruit.

Lunch   Quick Chicken or Turkey Rice Soup* and a side salad with butter lettuce.

Dinner   In a restaurant, order baked or broiled fish with vegetables and a small green salad.

Day 5

Breakfast   Omelette with baby shrimp and sautéed scallions and spinach.

Lunch   Salmon or halibut fish patty (see "Specialty Foods" in appendix B), mushroom and green bean sauté, rice, and a small green salad.

Dinner   Pan Fried Swordfish,* steamed cauliflower and broccoli, and rice.

Day 6

Breakfast   Breakfast Scramble* with diced turkey.

Lunch   Wonderful Whatever Salad* with leftover diced turkey.

Dinner   Wonderful Baked Chicken Breasts,* Green Bean and Mushroom Stir-Fry,* rice, and a small green salad.

Day 7

Breakfast   Breakfast Scramble* using diced chicken and small amounts of the Green Bean and Mushroom Stir-Fry,* and rice from last evening's dinner.

Lunch   Tuna salad with salad greens.

Dinner   Baked Shrimp and Scallops,* or your choice of rice or vegetable, stir-fried.

Beverages, Snacks, and Desserts

Often people stray from a diet when choosing beverages, snacks, and desserts. Here are some suggestions to keep things simple, and to keep you on the Anti-Inflammation Syndrome Diet Plan.

For cold beverages, stick with sparkling mineral or still waters and a wedge of lemon, lime, or orange. Many sparkling mineral waters, such as Gerolsteiner, have substantial calcium and magnesium levels—good for your health. For hot beverages, a herbal tea or a green tea is a good choice.

For snacks, it is best to stick with unsalted raw or roasted nuts. You can make your own blend of nuts and seeds that is probably superior to any commercial trail mix. Use almonds, pistachios, pumpkin seeds, macadamias, sunflower seeds, and organic raisins. You can also adapt a Moroccan appetizer by eating a couple of dates or figs with half a dozen raw almonds.

For desserts, one of the issues is not eating too much—a problem when you make or bake a dessert at home. It may be better to buy small amounts of "healthy" dessert items. Some possibilities include small amounts of Earthsong Cranberry-Orange and Apple-Walnut Whole Food Bars (www.earthsongwholefoods.com), Jennie's Coconut Macaroons (www.redmillfarms.com) bars, Nutiva Flax & Raisin bars (www.nutiva.com), and Hadley date rolls with almonds (www.hadley dates.com). Another possibility is a Van's apple-cinnamon toaster waffle, with almond butter or banana slices and powdered cinnamon.

PART III

The Anti-Inflammation Syndrome Supplement Plan

CHAPTER 8

Good Fats That Rev Up Your Body's Natural Anti-Inflammatories

—ɯ—

QUIZ 3

What Nutritional Supplements Do You Take?

Taking individual supplements indicates that you care about preserving your health, and taking specific anti-inflammatory supplements suggests that you are already trying to prevent or reverse an inflammatory disorder.

Do not include any supplements found in multivitamins or any other type of once-a-day supplement. The questions refer only to stand-alone supplements.

Do you take any supplements identified as fish oil, salmon oil, omega-3, EPA, DHA, or GLA?

Add 2 points _____

Do you take vitamin E supplements?

Add 2 points _____

Do you take vitamin C supplements?

Add 1 point _____

Do you take glucosamine or chondroitin supplements?

Add 1 point _____

Do you take devil's claw, green tea, Pycnogenol, grape seed extract, or quercetin supplements?

Add 1 point _____

Do you take herbal supplements such as St. John's wort, ginseng, ginkgo, or any other?

Add 1 point _____

Your score on quiz 3: _____

Initial interpretation and ranking:

0 Low. You do not take any anti-inflammation supplements, either because you do not need them or because you are not aware of them.

1–3 Moderate. You take some anti-inflammation supplements, which offer some protection.

4–8 High. You take numerous anti-inflammation supplements, suggesting that you are trying to reverse a chronic inflammatory condition.

Please note your quiz 1 score: _____ and ranking _____

Please note your quiz 2 score: _____ and ranking _____

Please note your quiz 3 score: _____ and ranking _____

—៣—

How to Interpret the Results of all Three Quizzes

High or very high on quiz 1 (page 14): You likely have considerable inflammation. The higher the score, the higher your level of inflammation.

High or very high on quiz 2 (page 61) *but not quiz 1:* You are at risk for developing inflammatory diseases in the coming years. This would be a good time to bolster your long-term health.

High or very high on both *quiz 1 and quiz 2:* You likely have a high level of inflammation. The reason is probably that you are eating too many pro-inflammatory foods. You would do well to go on the Anti-Inflammation Syndrome Diet Plan and take steps to improve your long-term health.

High or very high on quiz 1 but not quiz 2: You probably have adopted a very good diet, but may have to further fine-tune your diet and supplement program.

Factoring In Your Anti-Inflammatory Supplements

High on quiz 3: You are already taking some important supplements that can reduce your risk of inflammation.

High or very high on quizzes 1 and 3: You may need to take different supplements or increase their dosage.

High or very high on quizzes 2 and 3: You will have to work on improving your diet.

High or very high on quizzes 1, 2, and 3: You likely have a high level of inflammation, but you are only taking supplements instead of taking supplements *and* improving your diet. To improve your health, you must focus on *both* diet and supplements.

High or very high on quizzes 1 or 2 but low on quiz 3: You have been or are at high risk of chronic inflammation. You should take anti-inflammatory supplements.

Healthy oils play a pivotal role in controlling and reversing inflammation because they contain highly concentrated amounts of specific anti-inflammatory nutrients. Chief among these highly beneficial nutrients are omega-3 fatty acids found in fish oils; gamma-linolenic acid; and olive oil.

A wholesome diet, such as the one recommended in this book, provides ample quantities of these oils. However, you may want extra amounts of them to either jump-start your body's anti-inflammatory activities or to reverse health problems. You can buy omega-3 fatty acids, and gamma-linolenic acid in capsule form. Even though olive oil is a food product, not a supplement that comes in capsule form, this chapter discusses all three of these oils because they work together in the body to stem inflammation. Using generous amounts of olive oil in your cooking is a way to supplement your diet with extra amounts of it.

Anita: Fish Oil for Lower Blood Pressure

Anita was a widowed single mother who looked much older than her thirty-six years. The pressures of working and mothering three young children forced her to stop making home-cooked meals in favor of burgers, fries, pizzas, and quick-energy foods such as candy bars and soft drinks. At the end of each day she would collapse in bed, exhausted and drained.

Over two years Anita had gained thirty pounds and was now experiencing frequent headaches and suffering joint pain in her hips, shoulders, and hands. Her medical doctor prescribed ibuprofen, and a rheumatologist told her she had some (but not all) of the signs of lupus erythematosus. She was developing stomach pain from the ibuprofen, and medication for the lupuslike symptoms caused double vision. In addition, Anita's blood pressure had risen to 190/100 and her blood sugar was more than 240, clearly in the diabetic range. These clinical findings led to additional prescriptions for hypertensive and glucose-lowering medications.

A friend recommended that Anita consult with Judy A. Hutt, N.D., a naturopathic physician in Tucson, Arizona. After a workup Hutt asked Anita to eat a simple, wholesome diet similar to the Anti-Inflammation Syndrome Diet Plan. Anita began eating more fish, chicken, turkey, and vegetables, while avoiding processed foods, soft drinks, coffee, and dairy products. Hutt also asked her to take several anti-inflammatory supplements, including fish oil capsules (1,000 mg twice daily), as well as ginger, turmeric, and bromelain.

Anita's response was dramatic. After three weeks she had lost ten pounds and her glucose had normalized, enabling her to stop taking the glucose-lowering medications. Her pain, swelling, and stiffness decreased considerably, and her energy levels began increasing. At a six-week follow-up visit Anita had lost a total of eighteen pounds, and her blood pressure was normal, so she was able to stop taking the hypertensive medications. In addition, her joint pain was almost entirely gone, flaring up only when she went off her diet of simple, wholesome foods. Anita no longer had a need to take cortisone drugs for her lupuslike symptoms. Her headaches were gone, her energy levels were better, and she actually looked younger.

Omega-3 Fish Oils

As you read in chapter 3, the omega-3 family of fatty acids forms the building blocks of many of the body's natural anti-inflammatory compounds. Fish oil supplements, which are typically produced from salmon oil, are especially rich in eicosapentaenoic acid (EPA) and docosahexaenoic acid (DHA). Although both fatty acids are essential for health, EPA plays a more important role in the body's defenses against inflammation.

The advantage of taking fish oil or salmon oil capsules is simple: your body does not have to go through the many steps involved in converting alpha-linolenic acid (found in leafy green vegetables and flaxseed) to EPA and DHA. By taking capsules, you can leapfrog these steps and the potential bottlenecks that interfere with the conversion and help your body rapidly convert EPA to inflammation-suppressing eicosanoids.

Although you will read more about rheumatoid arthritis and osteoarthritis in later chapters, these two conditions serve as excellent examples of how fish oils can benefit your health. Numerous studies have documented that diets high in either fish or fish oils improve the balance of fatty acids in tissues, raising levels of anti-inflammatory and lowering amounts of pro-inflammatory substances.

More than two thousand studies on omega-3 fatty acids have been published in medical journals, adding up to a wealth of persuasive data, and many studies have found that supplements and omega-3 rich foods can significantly reduce levels of several inflammation-promoting compounds in people: thromboxane B_2, prostaglandin E_2, interleukin-1, and C-reactive protein. In a very real sense, fish oils snuff out many of the matches of inflammation.

This anti-inflammatory effect of fish oils has been demonstrated over and over again. For example, in a Scottish study, researchers asked sixty-four men and women with rheumatoid arthritis to take daily fish oil capsules, containing a little more than 1.7 grams of EPA and 1 gram of DHA or a placebo (dummy pill) daily. After three months many of the patients taking the fish oil capsules benefited from reduced pain and were able to lower their intake of nonsteroidal anti-inflammatory drugs (NSAIDs). By the end of the year-long study, 40 percent of the patients taking fish oil capsules had been able to lower or eliminate their NSAIDs, reducing their risk of drug-related side effects.

Fish oils actually help rebuild articular cartilage. Bruce Caterson, Ph.D., of Cardiff University, Wales, led a team of molecular biologists who discovered specifically why fish oils reduce inflammation and inhibit the breakdown of cartilage, one of the characteristics of osteoarthritis. Caterson first determined that chondrocytes, one of the key types of cells forming cartilage, readily absorbed alpha-linolenic acid (the parent omega-3 fatty acid) and displaced other fatty acids in the process. The same thing happened when he grew chondrocytes with EPA and DHA. But significantly, all of the omega-3 fatty acids deactivated "aggrecanases," a family of enzymes known to break down cartilage. The omega-3 fatty acids also stopped the genetic programming that increased levels of pro-inflammatory compounds, including interleukin-1 (IL-1), tumor necrosis factor alpha (TNFa), and cyclooxygenase-2 (Cox-2).

—ഗ—

Benefits of Omega-3 Fish Oils

- Reduce inflammation
- Natural, mild blood thinner
- Help maintain heart rhythm
- Reduce blood pressure
- Lower triglycerides
- Slow proliferation of cancer cells
- Improve mood disorders

—ഗ—

Fish Oils Protect the Heart

Early Arctic explorers made note of the rarity of coronary artery disease in Eskimos, despite their consumption of a high-fat and high-cholesterol diet. It wasn't until 1973 that two Danish researchers compared the diets of Arctic Eskimos to that of Greenland Eskimos, who ate diets similar to other Danes. The Greenland Eskimos, who consumed more saturated fat and cholesterol from meat and dairy products, had a higher rate of heart disease.

Since then, many other studies have confirmed the heart-protective effect of omega-3 fatty acids, especially EPA. For example, a twenty-five-year study of dietary and health data of almost thirteen thousand men in seven countries found that elevated blood cholesterol levels were associated with heart disease only in areas where intake of omega-3 and omega-9 fatty acids were low. A separate study of four hundred people, conducted by Michel de Lorgeril, M.D., of Saint-Étienne, France, found that adoption of a Mediterranean-style diet can greatly lower the likelihood of a second heart attack. Lorgeril and his colleagues asked patients to follow a Mediterranean-style diet, high in fish, vegetables, and olive oil, or to continue eating their usual diet. People eating the Mediterranean-style diet were 50 to 70 percent less likely to have a second heart attack during the four-year study. They also had less than half the risk of developing cancer or dying from any natural cause.

In 2001 Canadian researchers reported that Eskimos who adhere to their traditional diet experience relatively little heart disease. The Nunavik Inuit of Québec eat a diet that includes both a traditional diet, consisting of fish and marine mammals, along with some Western refined foods. They maintain high blood levels of EPA and DHA—and have half the incidence of death from heart disease compared with other residents of Québec.

Fish oils have at least two other cardiovascular benefits: they are mild and natural blood thinners, and they help maintain a normal heart rhythm. Arrhythmias are erratic heartbeats that can go out of control, leading to ventricular tachycardia and cardiac arrest. Experiments by Alexander Leaf, M.D., of Harvard Medical School, found that supplemental EPA and DHA could prevent arrhythmias and ventricular fibrillations. A separate study of more than eight hundred people conducted by David S. Siscovick, M.D., of the University of Washington, found that one fish meal weekly reduced the risk of cardiac arrest by half, compared with people who ate no fish at all. Five ounces of salmon contain about 7.5 grams of omega-3 fatty acids.

Fish Oils May Reduce Cancer Risk

The health benefits of fish oils extend to general protection against cancer. Bruce N. Ames, Ph.D., an eminent cell biologist at the University of California, Berkeley, has pointed out that 30 percent of cancers result from chronic inflammation and chronic infections (and infections cause inflammation).

In fact, large amounts of omega-6 fatty acids, in the form of linoleic acid-rich corn and safflower oils, promote the proliferation of breast and prostate cancers. In contrast, fish oils clearly prevent and slow the growth of cancers. Corn oil has an omega-6 to omega-3 ratio of 60:1, and safflower oil a ratio of 77:1—far from the evolutionary balance of 1:1.

Human studies are consistent with animal studies showing that omega-3 fish oils protect against cancer. Paul Terry, Ph.D., and his colleagues at the Karolinska Institute in Stockholm, tracked the health of more than six thousand male twins who were, on average, in their mid-fifties when the study began. Terry found that men who regularly ate fish had one-half to one-third the risk of prostate cancer, compared with those who ate no fish.

Other Anti-Inflammatory Benefits of Fish Oils

Evidence of the broader anti-inflammatory effects of fish and fish oil supplements comes from other types of medical research, such as on asthma and Crohn's disease, a type of inflammatory bowel disease. For example, an Australian study found that children with asthma were half as likely to consume fish rich in omega-3 fatty acids. As little as one fish meal per week was enough to reduce the likelihood of asthma.

In a separate study, described in the *New England Journal of Medicine,* researchers gave either fish oil supplements or placebos to seventy-eight patients with Crohn's disease. The fish oil capsules provided about 600 mg of EPA and 300 mg of DHA daily. After one year 59 percent of the patients taking fish oil capsules were still in remission, more than twice that of the placebo group.

How to Buy and Use Fish Oil Supplements

There are so many omega-3 fish oil supplements on the market that it is often confusing to choose a brand. If you can, opt for a brand from fish caught in relatively pollution-free waters. Doing so will lower your likelihood of consuming extra mercury or other toxins. Some companies identify the source of their fish oils, such as Norwegian salmon.

Most fish oil supplements contain roughly three-fifths EPA and two-fifths DHA. If you want a high-EPA supplement use Omega-Brite, which contains 90 percent EPA and 10 percent DHA. To enhance the anti-inflammatory effects of omega-3 fish oils take gamma-linolenic acid supplements. (See the following section.) DHA supplements made from algae may not have the anti-inflammatory effect of EPA, but they may provide other health benefits, such as improving memory.

Flaxseed is a rich nonanimal source of alpha-linolenic acid, and flaxseed oil capsules are sometimes recommended as a source of omega-3 fatty acids. While flaxseed is indeed an excellent source of alpha-linolenic acid, many people have difficulty converting it to EPA and DHA, which would limit its usefulness as a supplement.

Dosage: For prevention of inflammatory disorders, take 1 gram of omega-3 fish oil capsules daily. If you have a form of arthritis, take at least 3 grams daily of omega-3 fish oils. If you never eat fish, you may want to take at least 5 grams of fish oils daily. In addition, take 400 IU of natural vitamin E daily, which will protect the fish oils from free-radical damage.

Side effects: Fish oil supplements have been shown to lower blood levels of triglyceride, a fat associated with an increased risk of coronary artery disease, but sometimes to raise cholesterol levels slightly. In addition, the blood-thinning effect of fish oils may be magnified if you take several other blood thinners, including vitamin E, ginkgo, or Coumadin.

Ask your physician to monitor you, especially if you are taking Coumadin, a prescription anticoagulant drug.

Nelda: Fish Oil to Relieve Pain

Back in 1980, at age sixty-three, Nelda was displaying all the signs of rheumatoid arthritis. Her fingers, which hurt all the time, were becoming red and deformed. She was taking prescription pain relievers six to eight times daily, and her family physician was suggesting that it might be better to replace her right knee and left hip joints. Nelda was also taking nitroglycerin for her heart and a blood pressure-lowering medication.

She figured there had to be an alternative, so she visited Hugh D. Riordan, M.D., president of the Center for the Improvement of Human Functioning International in Wichita, Kansas. Laboratory tests showed Nelda sensitive to some of her favorite foods, specifically dairy products and white potatoes, which she immediately stopped eating. She also began taking a number of anti-inflammatory supplements, including fish oils and antioxidant vitamins.

In less than a year Nelda was virtually pain-free and had regained flexibility in her fingers. She stood straight and no longer needed a cane or a walker. For the next twenty years Nelda remained active, healthier in her seventies and eighties than in her sixties.

Gamma-Linolenic Acid

Gamma-linolenic acid, or GLA, is part of the omega-6 family, but it behaves more like an anti-inflammatory omega-3 fatty acid. GLA is found in seeds, and nearly all supplemental forms are derived from borage, evening primrose, or black currant seeds. It constitutes about 20 percent of borage seed oil, 15 to 19 percent of black currant seed oil, and 9 percent of evening primrose seed oil. If you have been consuming vegetable oils such as corn, safflower, or soy, do not assume that your body has been converting its linoleic acid to GLA. Foods high in these oils are often high in trans fatty acids, which interfere with the conversion process.

As with fish oil EPA and DHA supplements, GLA supplements leapfrog several steps and quickly raise blood levels of GLA. GLA boosts production of DGLA, the immediate precursor of prostaglandin E_1, which suppresses inflammation.

Several human trials have found GLA supplements to greatly benefit patients with rheumatoid arthritis; they also seem to help restore more normal immune responses. In one investigation, Robert Zurier, M.D., of the University of Massachusetts at Worcester, treated thirty-seven patients with rheumatoid arthritis and inflamed joints. He gave them either 1.4 grams of GLA or placebos daily. After twenty-four weeks both physicians and patients noted significant reductions in symptoms. The number of tender joints among patients taking GLA was reduced by 36 percent, and the overall score on tests measuring tender joints declined by 45 percent. In addition, the number of swollen joints decreased by 28 percent, and the patients' overall score for swollen joints fell by 41 percent. Some people benefited far more than did others, but that is frequently the case with nutritional supplements. It is likely that better responses would have occurred with a broader supplement regimen, but the study was designed to test GLA only.

In another study Zurier doubled the dosage of GLA, giving fifty-six patients either 2.8 grams daily of the supplement or placebos for six months. This higher dosage resulted in significant improvements—at least a 25 percent improvement in four of eight measures of rheumatoid arthritis severity. For a second six-month period, Zurier gave GLA to all of the patients, and improvements were noted across the board. The group originally given GLA continued to improve over the course of a year, with more than three-fourths of the patients benefiting from improvements in their arthritis symptoms.

How to Buy and Use GLA Supplements

Virtually all supplemental GLA is derived from evening primrose, borage, or black currant seed oils. Many of the GLA supplements sold are actually labeled as "evening primrose," "borage seed oil," or "black currant seed oil," with the actual quantity of GLA listed in fine print on the back of the label. As you might expect, each type of oil has its proponent, often because of financial interests.

Although the concentration of GLA is highest in borage seed oil and lowest in evening primrose oil, it is more important to identify the specific quantity of GLA per capsule (or per several capsules). All of this information is on the label. Once you have identified the quantity of GLA per daily serving, calculate its cost and compare it in similar fashion to other GLA supplements.

Dosage: The dosage of GLA used in arthritis studies ranges from 1.4 to 2.8 grams daily—again, this is the dosage of GLA, not the total weight of oil in the capsules. As always, read supplement labels carefully. For example, a product may contain 1,000 mg of black current seed oil but only 150 mg of GLA per two capsules. Depending on the brand, 2.8 grams of GLA might translate to more than twenty capsules daily! You can likely benefit from lower dosages of GLA if you take them with other supplements, such as fish oils and vitamin E.

Side effects: Rare.

Victor: Olympic Nutrition

Søren Mavrogenis, the physiotherapist for the Danish Olympic team, began recommending a combination of omega-3 fatty acids, gamma-linolenic acid, and antioxidants in 1996. At the time he had been treating the inflamed knee of a female rower but had not been able to help her. Because of the side effects of nonsteroidal anti-inflammatory drugs (NSAIDs), Mavrogenis was reluctant to recommend them for long-term use.

Mavrogenis's conversations with health writer Bjørn Falck Madsen and a researcher at a Scandinavian vitamin company led to a specific supplement regimen. The rower started taking the supplements and was able to resume rowing within a few weeks. One success led to another, and today Mavrogenis routinely uses a combination of omega-3 fatty acids, gamma-linolenic acid, and antioxidants (brand name Bio-Sport), along with deep muscle massage, to treat chronic overuse and inflammatory disorders. About one-third of his clinic's patients are elite athletes.

One of Mavrogenis's patients has been Victor A. Feddersen, a world champion rower and Olympic gold medalist in 1996. During training and competition, Feddersen suffered inflammatory injuries to his elbows. In the past he had to take a break from training and use NSAIDs. But for the past several years Feddersen has taken fatty acid and antioxidant supplements while also undergoing Mavrogenis's deep-muscle massage. It has made a big difference. He responds quickly to the supplements and has been able to continue training while recuperating.

Other Danish Olympic athletes have benefited similarly with a variety of inflammatory injuries, including those of the shoulders, arms, legs, and Achilles' heal. In general, inflammation subsides about a month after starting the supplements, but some people have responded within a week, while others take several months.

Olive Oil

Think of olive oil as one of the tastiest "supplements" you can eat. A common constituent of Greek and Italian diets, olive oil is rich in oleic acid, an omega-9 fatty acid. Many of the heart-healthy benefits of the traditional Mediterranean diet have been attributed to its abundant use of olive oil. Although other aspects of the diet (e.g., fruits, vegetables, and fish) are healthful, scientific studies have found olive oil to possess impressive anti-inflammatory properties in its own right.

Diets high in olive oil appear to reduce the likelihood of developing rheumatoid arthritis. Christos S. Mantzoros, M.D., D.Sc., of Harvard Medical School, and researchers from the Athens Medical School, found that consumption of olive oil was associated with a 61 percent lower risk of having rheumatoid arthritis. In another study, Parveen Yaqoob, Ph.D., a researcher at the University of Southampton, England, asked healthy middle-age men to eat either a conventional diet or one high in olive oil for two months. The men eating extra olive oil had a specific type of "adhesion molecule" that was 20 percent less active. This adhesion molecule, known as ICAM-1, sustains inflammatory and allergic reactions. By reducing the activity of adhesion molecules, olive oil tempers inflammatory reactions.

How to Buy and Use Olive Oil

As was discussed in chapter 6, the best varieties of olive oil are "extra virgin," because they are produced during the first mechanical pressing of olives. Pure or classic olive oil also is made from the first pressing, but it is slightly more acidic and can tolerate higher cooking temperatures. Light olive oil has been filtered to reduce its natural fragrance; it has no fewer calories than the other forms.

You should use olive oil exclusively or nearly exclusively as your cooking oil. Grapeseed oil also is rich in omega-9 fatty acids, but it is often produced through chemical extraction. Some mechanically pressed grapeseed oil is available, but you have to search for it in stores. While grapeseed oil is tolerant of very high temperatures, olive oil is still the preferred oil at home and in restaurants.

Other major food sources of omega-9 fatty acids are avocados and macadamia nuts. Both foods have been shown to reduce blood cholesterol levels, though their health benefits may be partly related to other nutrients.

Dosage: While there is no specific recommended amount, use extra-virgin olive oil liberally when cooking at home.

Side effects: Rare.

In this chapter you have read how "good" fats can help restore a normal inflammatory response and, in doing so, reduce symptoms of rheumatoid arthritis, osteoarthritis, and other inflammatory disorders. These fats also can lower blood pressure and lower your risk of heart disease and cancer. In the following chapter you will learn how vitamin E is now being recognized as the leading anti-inflammatory vitamin.

CHAPTER 9

Vitamin E to Extinguish the Flames of Inflammation

Long known to reduce the risk of coronary artery (heart) disease, vitamin E has recently been shown, in scientific studies with people, to possess significant anti-inflammatory properties. More than any other single nutrient, vitamin E can significantly reduce a variety of key indicators and promoters of inflammation.

For example, vitamin E lowers levels of C-reactive protein and interleukin-6 and reduces the activity of various types of "adhesion molecules" that promote inflammation throughout the body. In fact, vitamin E may be the single most important nutrient for lowering CRP levels. It should therefore not come as a surprise that, in addition to reducing the risk of heart disease, vitamin E is beneficial in Alzheimer's disease, arthritis, allergies, cancer, and many other inflammatory diseases. This chapter will focus on its emerging role as the premier anti-inflammatory vitamin.

Dr. Kunin and Susan: Antioxidants for Health

Years ago, Richard Kunin, M.D., of San Francisco, California, described himself as a "nasal neurotic." He had asthma, was allergic to dogs and cats, and sneezed literally a hundred times a day. He became interested in nutritional medicine, cured himself of all of his nasal and respiratory problems, and has gone on to become one of the most original and eclectic thinkers in "orthomolecular medicine," which focuses on using nutrition to achieve optimal health.

One patient, Susan, had high blood pressure much of her adult life but opted not to treat it medically. By her late sixties she had undergone a triple coronary-artery bypass. She consulted Dr. Kunin after repeated attacks of angina (heart pain), arrhythmias after exercising, muscle aches, postoperative memory loss, bronchitis, and coughing. Memory loss is common after bypass surgery, and Susan had difficulty recalling her recent medical history.

Based on Susan's medical history and laboratory tests, Kunin diagnosed her high prothrombin (blood clotting) activity and that it was likely the result of a genetic propensity toward excessive blood clotting. He also felt that Susan's muscle aches were the result of the statin drug interfering with her body's production of coenzyme Q_{10}, a vitaminlike substance needed for energy production in muscle cells.

Susan also had an acute sense of smell, which Kunin recognized as a likely sign of chemical sensitivity. The most likely culprit was Susan's forced-air gas furnace. Such furnaces, as well as gas stoves, release burned hydrocarbons into the air, and sensitive people react to these compounds. Kunin recommended that she replace the filter and update her heating system.

Kunin then developed an antioxidant and anticoagulant regimen for Susan to follow, based in part on the fact that vitamin antioxidants also have blood-thinning properties. Use of bromelain supplements served as a natural way to reduce blood viscosity (caused by excessive fibrin), as did use of small oral amounts of heparin, an anticoagulant drug. Heparin, Kunin explained, has anticoagulant effects when taken orally (not just by injection) but does not interfere with vitamin K metabolism the way Coumadin does.

Because Susan had large numbers of "activated" blood platelet cells, Kunin also recommended that she take supplements of the herb Ginkgo biloba, which inhibits platelet activity. Among the other supplements were B vitamins, vitamin C, vitamin E, alpha-lipoic acid, and the amino acid arginine.

Susan's health has improved considerably. Her blood pressure has been reduced, and she no longer has arrhythmias or muscle aches.

Vitamin E and Heart Disease

The role of vitamin E in preventing and reversing cardiovascular diseases was first reported by Canadian physicians Evan V. Shute, M.D., Wilfrid Shute, M.D., and their colleagues in the 1940s. At that time no one understood the role of inflammation in cardiovascular diseases, and C-reactive protein had not yet been discovered. Indeed, until the 1990s, the medical establishment was generally skeptical that a single vitamin could play a pivotal role in reversing heart disease.

Today, with a clearer picture of the role of inflammation in heart disease and good documentation for the anti-inflammatory and heart-protective role of vitamin E, the early successes of the Shute brothers are better understood. Certainly, vitamin E has important health roles beyond that of just a mild and safe anti-inflammatory nutrient. It is the body's principal fat-soluble antioxidant and, as such, blocks free-radical oxidation to cholesterol, which stimulates inflammation and is one of the initiators of heart disease. As an anticoagulant, vitamin E helps prevent abnormal blood clots. It also inhibits the proliferation of "smooth muscle" cells in coronary arteries, which contributes to the narrowing of blood vessels.

The striking benefits of vitamin E in preventing and reversing heart disease have been confirmed by several recent human trials. The most impressive study, conducted in England and published in the highly respected journal *Lancet*, involved two thousand patients with heart disease. About half were given either 400 or 800 IU of natural vitamin E, while the others received placebos. After an average of eighteen months the group taking vitamin E had only one-fourth the number of nonfatal heart attacks as did the placebo group. Although the vitamin E group experienced slightly more fatal heart attacks, a subsequent analysis of the data found that almost all of these deaths were among people who failed to take their vitamin E supplements.

It is rare, however, for biomedical studies to be 100 percent consistent in their results, and this is true with vitamin E studies. For example, one recent study found no benefits from taking the vitamin, which has made many physicians reconsider their use of vitamin E. Yet in a recent analysis of the five largest studies of vitamin E and heart disease, Ishwarlal "Kenny" Jialal, M.D., a cardiologist and antioxidant researcher at the University of Texas Southwestern Medical Center, Dallas, noted that four of the largest human trials supported the use of vitamin E and the fifth had troubling design problems.

Roberta: Natural Anti-Inflammatories for Crohn's Disease

Shari Lieberman, Ph.D., who has been a clinical nutritionist for more than twenty years, explains it this way: if you were a child and told your mother that your stomach hurt, she would ask what you had eaten. Lieberman can't understand why many physicians don't do the same when it comes to gastrointestinal disorders such as Crohn's disease.

In 1986 Roberta consulted with Lieberman about a diagnosis of Crohn's disease. She was fourteen years old and previously had seen several gastrointestinal specialists. By this time Roberta was taking two prescription anti-inflammatory drugs, prednisone and sulfasalazine, but was still experiencing vomiting and diarrhea and had lost weight. Her physician had recently suggested surgery to remove the lower portion of her ileum, part of the small intestine.

After an evaluation, Lieberman suspected that gluten intolerance was at the core of Roberta's problems and that dairy was likely a contributing factor. In gluten-sensitive people this protein triggers an autoimmune reaction that often leads to wide-ranging food sensitivities. Roberta was also under considerable stress related to family issues, and Lieberman made a referral to help Roberta cope with these problems.

In terms of diet, Lieberman recommended that Roberta avoid all food containing gluten—chiefly wheat, rye, and barley—as well as dairy. She also suggested a number of supplements. Among them were betonite clay and psyllium supplements, both of which add bulk without being a laxative. This nonlaxative effect was important to avoid further diarrhea. Lieberman also suggested fish oils for their anti-inflammatory properties and a number of antioxidants, including 1,000 mg of vitamin C and 1,200 of natural vitamin E, plus a high-potency multivitamin/multimineral supplement.

Within two weeks Roberta's diarrhea ceased and blood stopped appearing in her stools. After six months her physician saw no further need for the prescription drugs. The only times symptoms of Crohn's disease have reappeared were when Roberta has been under extreme psychological stress. She has been in remission for more than fifteen years.

How Vitamin E Reduces Inflammation

The details of how coronary artery disease begins are complex, and sometimes, like the chicken-and-egg story, it is difficult to discern exactly what step comes before another. It is likely that many events are occurring simultaneously, including inflammation of the arteries.

During the 1990s it became clear that high levels of the low-density lipoprotein (LDL) form of cholesterol increased the risk of heart disease. Basically, the idea is that LDL appears to be neutral until it is oxidized, or damaged by free radicals.

It has become fashionable to describe LDL as the "bad" form of cholesterol, but this is a misnomer because it is not inherently unhealthy. LDL is necessary for transporting vitamin E and other fat-soluble nutrients through the blood. In other words, these antioxidants should normally be present in LDL and prevent its oxidation. LDL oxidation occurs when dietary vitamin E and other antioxidants are insufficient, or when there is a large amount of cholesterol relative to vitamin E.

Free radicals stimulate and amplify inflammatory reactions through a number of mechanisms. For example, free radicals activate some of the genes involved in inflammation. They also turn on a variety of adhesion molecules, which, as the term suggests, encourage white blood cells to stick to normal cells, such as the endothelial cells that line blood vessel walls.

Vitamin E blocks the inflammatory process in a variety of ways:

- As an antioxidant, it quenches free radicals, thus reducing their ability to stimulate abnormal inflammatory responses.
- Vitamin E inhibits at least two transcription factors, preventing the activation of some of the genes involved in inflammation.
- It turns off a variety of adhesion molecules, helping to keep inflammatory reactions from going out of control.
- The vitamin blocks one of the omega-6 pathways (5-lipoxygenase) involved in making inflammation-causing substances.
- Vitamin E prevents the oxidation of LDL cholesterol, thus discouraging white blood cells from migrating toward the arteries.
- It is a mild cyclooxygenase-2 (Cox-2) inhibitor. By quenching peroxynitrite, a type of free radical, vitamin E reduces levels of proinflammatory prostaglandin E_2, which subsequently lowers Cox-2 activity.
- Vitamin E supplements can lower CRP levels in many people by 30 to 50 percent.

This remarkable CRP-lowering effect has so far been demonstrated in two well-designed human trials. In one, Jane E. Upritchard, Ph.D., and her colleagues at the University of Otago, New Zealand, tested the effects of three antioxidants on fifty-seven people with adult-onset diabetes. The supplements included 800 IU of natural vitamin E, 500 mg of vitamin C, and tomato juice (rich in lycopene) daily for four weeks. Upritchard reported in *Diabetes Care* that the vitamin E supplements, but not other antioxidants, lowered CRP levels by half!

In the other study Ishwarlal Jialal, M.D., asked seventy-two subjects, including some healthy and others with diabetes or heart disease, to take 1,200 IU of natural vitamin E daily for three months. Each of the three groups had decreases in CRP by an average of 30 percent and IL-6 by 50 percent.

—⁓—

C-Reactive Protein: The Current Standard for Measuring Inflammation

C-reactive protein (CRP), found in trace amounts in healthy people, has quickly emerged as the leading marker of systemic (or bodywide) inflammation. It is easy and inexpensive to test for, and you should ask your physician to measure your levels. You'll be hearing more and more about it: people with elevated CRP levels are 4½ times more likely to have a heart attack, compared with people who have normal levels of the protein. Furthermore, a variety of serious diseases are associated with high blood levels of CRP.

The good news is that natural vitamin E supplements can lower CRP levels by 30 to 50 percent.

Normal high-sensitivity levels are less than 0.11 milligram per deciliter of blood (mg/dL). Moderate CRP levels, of 0.12 to 0.19 mg/dL, are a cause for concern, and high CRP levels are 0.20 to 1.50 mg/dL. However, CRP levels can go up to 400 to 500 mg/dL in seriously ill people.

CRP levels are elevated in many different diseases and conditions.

Heart disease. High CRP levels are a better indicator than total cholesterol, LDL cholesterol, or homocysteine in predicting the risk of a heart attack, as well as of death in the first month after coronary artery bypass surgery. CRP is present in lesions (commonly but incorrectly referred to as cholesterol deposits) that form on blood vessel walls but not on normal blood vessel walls. CRP also is strongly associated with the rupture of these lesions, which can lead to dangerous blood vessel clots.

Blood sugar disorders. Insulin resistance, Syndrome X, and diabetes are all associated with increased levels of CRP. This is significant because each of these conditions increases the risk of coronary artery disease.

Dental disease. People with periodontal disease also have elevated CRP levels. This elevation may be the result of chronic infection or inflammation of the gums. It may also reflect inadequate levels of antioxidants, which would promote healing.

Smoking. Tobacco smoke raises CRP levels, and some researchers have found that they remain elevated in ex-smokers.

Overweight and obesity. Being overweight increases CRP levels. The reason is that adipose cells, particularly those that form around the abdomen (belly), produce large amounts of IL-6 and CRP. The implications are significant: being fat is partly an inflammatory disorder, and body fat promotes inflammation. This may be part of the reason why being overweight increases the risk of diabetes, heart disease, and other disorders. CRP levels are generally elevated in overweight children as well as adults.

Alzheimer's disease. High CRP levels also have been identified in patients with Alzheimer's disease, which researchers increasingly view as an inflammatory brain disorder.

Cancer. Many cancer patients have elevated CRP levels, which reflect an undercurrent of inflammation. This systemic inflammation may contribute to the breakdown of tissues and increase the risk of the cancer spreading.

Arthritis. People with "traditional" inflammatory diseases, such as arthritis and asthma, commonly have elevated levels of CRP or other markers of abnormally high inflammation.

—◠◡◠—

Vitamin E and Rheumatoid Arthritis

Consistent with the anti-inflammatory properties of vitamin E are clinical studies showing that it can reduce inflammation and pain in patients with rheumatoid arthritis. The first study, published in *Annals of the Rheumatic Diseases* in 1997, described how a team of British and German researchers treated forty-two patients with either about 1,800 IU (900 IU twice daily) of vitamin E or placebos daily for twelve weeks. The subjects kept a daily diary describing their early-morning stiffness, evening pain, and pain after routine daily activities.

On average, arthritis pain decreased by about half among patients taking vitamin E supplements. Furthermore, more patients taking vitamin E improved compared with those taking placebos—60 percent versus 32 percent. The researchers suggested that vitamin E might work, in part, by quenching nitric oxide, a free radical involved in the sensation of pain.

A second study, published in the German medical journal *Arznei-mittel Forschung/Drug Research* in 2001, tested three treatments on a group of thirty patients with rheumatoid arthritis: one entailed pharmaceutical treatment, another was pharmaceutical treatment plus a modest antioxidant supplement, and the other was pharmaceutical treatment plus 600 IU of vitamin E three times daily. Significantly, patients taking the antioxidants or the vitamin E noted tangible improvements during the first month of treatment. Those taking only the drug treatment did not report any benefits until the end of the second month. Patients taking the antioxidants or vitamin E had higher levels of glutathione peroxidase, a powerful antioxidant made by the body, and lower levels of free radicals.

—∭—

Talking Nutrition with Your Physician

If you are like many people, you have been frustrated when trying to discuss diet or supplements with your physician. All too often, doctors quickly and arrogantly dismiss their patients' questions on these subjects.

Why? Nobel laureate and vitamin advocate Linus Pauling, Ph.D., explained it this way: "If a doctor isn't 'up' on something, he's 'down' on it." That is *really* the case.

The truth is that most physicians don't know much about nutrition because medical schools have given the subject a very low priority. Medicine, as the name suggests, places greatest emphasis on pharmaceutical medicines and surgery. It's hard for many people, including physicians, to admit that they don't know much about a particular subject.

Physicians also can be as gullible as the rest of us, swayed by the limitations of their own training, pharmaceutical company advertising, and misleading articles that question the value of diet and vitamin supplements.

Nutritionally oriented physicians have suggested that the best way to talk about nutritional therapies with a skeptical doc is to be firm but non-confrontational. Physicians don't have a lot of time to keep up with their specialty, let alone delve into another one, such as nutrition. They may also have financial and therapeutic constraints imposed by a health maintenance organization (HMO), insurer, or even the other doctors in his office.

One approach might be to say something like: "Doctor, using vitamins and fatty acids to treat my inflammation appeals to me because they are safe and the evidence seems pretty solid. I would prefer not to treat myself so, as your patient, I would like you to take some time to seriously study some of the research in this area. I'll even loan you this book, which contains medical references at the back. Please do me a favor and take the time to look into this and work with me."

If that fails, you might have to change physicians to find one who is nutritionally oriented. This is easier than it used to be, and the names of several organizations making referrals to nutritionally oriented physicians are listed in appendix B. Most nutritionally oriented physicians are not part of HMOs, and insurers may reimburse for only some of their services. In other words, they work in a traditional fee-for-service arrangement, so you will have to pay by cash, check, or credit card. This may be more expensive, but it will likely lead to a nutritional program, a doctor who takes a little more time with you, and better care.

—∿—

Vitamin E and Nasal Allergies

Two studies have pointed to benefits from vitamin E in nasal and respiratory allergies. Andrew Fogarty, M.D., of the University of Nottingham, England, analyzed dietary data and blood levels of immunoglobulin E (IgE) from about twenty-five hundred people. IgE is an antibody produced in excessive amounts by people with asthma, rhinitis, and hay fever. Fogarty reported in *Lancet* that higher vitamin E intake was associated with lower levels of IgE. Each 1-mg increase in vitamin E intake, up to 7 mg (about 11 IU), was related to a 5.2 percent reduction in IgE levels.

This finding is consistent with animal research showing that vitamin E can lower IgE levels and, consequently, may lessen the symptoms of some allergies. One of those studies, using laboratory mice, found that supplemental vitamin E lowered blood levels of IgE as well as cytokines.

Based on all of these studies, you might think that vitamin E can suppress immunity and increase the risk of infections. However, the opposite appears to be true, suggesting that vitamin E plays a role in regulating normal immune responses. Simin Nikbin Meydani, D.V.M., Ph.D., of Tufts University, gave seventy-eight healthy seniors various amounts of vitamin E or placebos for eight months. She found that people taking 200 IU of vitamin E daily improved their immune response, measured by a viral or bacterial challenge in the skin, by an average of 65 percent. Levels of prostaglandin E_2 decreased, hinting that high levels of this pro-inflammatory substance interfere with the normal immune response to infection. Although the study was not intended to measure whether vitamin E reduced the number of infections, Meydani did find that patients taking vitamin E reported having 30 percent fewer colds than did the placebo group.

Vitamin E and Alzheimer's Disease

Research has shown that long-term use of anti-inflammatory medications such as nonsteroidal anti-inflammatory drugs (NSAIDs) can lower the risk of Alzheimer's disease and help maintain cognitive function in patients with the disease. However, NSAIDs pose serious side effects and do not address the root of the problem.

Hazardous free radicals, which go out of control when people fail to consume enough antioxidants, were implicated in the aging process back in 1954. Their role in damaging genes and cells is now generally accepted in medicine, and many Alzheimer's disease researchers believe that free radicals play a major role in the cognitive decline and behavioral changes characteristic of this disease.

For example, amyloid beta protein, which strangles brain cells in Alzheimer's disease, releases large numbers of free radicals that injure brain cells, according to research by Ashley I. Bush, M.D., Ph.D., a neurology researcher at Harvard Medical School. In an experiment with brain cells from rats, Allan Butterfield, Ph.D., a professor of chemistry at the University of Kentucky, Lexington, found that vitamin E prevented the formation of free radicals in brain cells and protected them from the toxic effects of amyloid beta protein. The benefits of vitamin E were demonstrated by Mary Sano, Ph.D., of Columbia University College of Physicians and Surgeons, New York, in a study of 342 patients with advanced Alzheimer's disease. Some of the patients received 2,000 IU of vitamin E (a hefty dose, not recommended for healthy people), while others received a drug or placebo for two years. This relatively short period of vitamin E supplementation delayed the onset of end-stage Alzheimer's disease by almost eight months.

At the time of this study, Sano considered only vitamin E's antioxidant effect against free radicals. However, research has shown that a variety of pro-inflammatory compounds congregate in the brain of patients with Alzheimer's disease. It is likely that vitamin E's anti-inflammatory properties also help prevent and slow the disease's progression. Meanwhile, Sano has begun a new study to determine whether large amounts of supplemental vitamin E might slow the progress of Alzheimer's disease in its earlier stages.

Optimizing the "Antioxidant Network"

You may obtain greater benefits by taking multiple antioxidants in addition to vitamin E. According to Lester Packer, Ph.D., of the University of California, Berkeley, antioxidants work best as a team. Antioxidants get used up rapidly fighting free radicals, but a diversity of antioxidants helps them regenerate to full strength. Many different antioxidants also help neutralize many different types of free radicals, with the result often being a faster recovery time.

For example, physicians at Loyola University Medical Center, Chicago, found that a combination of vitamins E and C reduced radiation proctitis—a type of rectal inflammation caused by radiation treatment. As another example, Italian researchers reported that hereditary pancreatitis, a painful recurring inflammation of the pancreas, could be reduced by a combination of vitamins E and C, selenium, and other antioxidants.

How to Take and Use Vitamin E

Vitamin E's impressive anti-inflammatory properties suggest that supplements would be beneficial in most and perhaps all inflammatory diseases, though its effect may be very subtle in some conditions. The food supply—even a diet built around whole foods—does not provide sufficient amounts of vitamin E, and most dietary vitamin E consists of the gamma tocopherol form, which has a limited role in human health.

Various binding and transport molecules select primarily the natural d-alpha tocopherol (or tocopheryl) form of the vitamin over all other natural and synthetic forms. To distinguish natural from synthetic vitamin E, you have to read the fine print on the label: "d-alpha . . ." refers to natural, and "dl-alpha . . ." refers to synthetic vitamin E. These two molecules are different. The natural form is absorbed twice as well in blood and tissues compared with the synthetic form, so do not buy synthetic vitamin E or any product where the source is ambiguous.

Good choices are d-alpha tocopheryl acetate, d-alpha tocopheryl succinate, d-alpha tocopherol with other mixed natural tocopherols, which would include a little beta and gamma tocopherol, or a mix of natural vitamin E tocopherols and tocotrienols. The mixed tocopherols most closely resemble how the vitamin occurs in nature, and at least gamma tocopherol may provide additional anti-inflammatory properties. Another option would be a supplement containing mixed natural vitamin E tocopherols and tocotrienols (a less well-known group of vitamin E molecules, but one that is gaining more recognition). Health and natural food stores tend to sell natural vitamin E products and generally have many choices, whereas pharmacies tend to sell synthetic vitamin E supplements. There are many excellent brands, but one of the most reliable is produced by J. R. Carlson Laboratories (888-234-5656; more details in appendix B).

Based on the research, a minimum of 200 IU of vitamin E daily is required to gain any significant health benefits; 400 IU (a small capsule) is a more ideal dosage. Some studies have used 800 IU and 1,200 IU daily, but the extra benefits do not appear to be worth the extra cost for most people. However, if you have a very high total cholesterol or LDL cholesterol level, 800 IU may certainly do a better job of preventing your cholesterol from being oxidized. It would also be important to drastically reduce your intake of cooking oils, except for olive oil.

In this chapter you have learned about the impressive anti-inflammatory properties of vitamin E. It lowers levels of CRP and many other pro-inflammatory compounds, and it reduces the risk of coronary artery disease. In addition, vitamin E supplements can, for many people, ease the symptoms of rheumatoid arthritis, allergies, and Alzheimer's disease. In the next chapter you will read about three nutrients that play a central role in maintaining and rebuilding tissues in the body.

CHAPTER 10

Glucosamine, Chondroitin, and Vitamin C to Rebuild Your Tissues

In the 1990s millions of people with osteoarthritis began taking supplements of two obscure dietary supplements, glucosamine and chondroitin. At the time of their initial popularity, glucosamine and chondroitin were supported by tantalizing evidence but limited clinical experience. The groundswell of interest in these supplements prompted physicians to conduct many clinical trials with people, which have confirmed that the supplements are effective in relieving pain *and* in restoring the cartilage pads that protect joints. Many of these studies also included vitamin C, an essential nutrient needed for the formation of cartilage and other tissue proteins.

This chapter will describe the recent research on glucosamine, chondroitin, and vitamin C. It begins with a brief overview of their roles in the formation of cartilage, then shifts to a discussion of the research, which is extraordinarily persuasive, on osteoarthritis. (Chapter 12 will discuss osteoarthritis in greater depth.) In a very real sense, these nutrients help hold us together, and supplements can help reinforce our health, slowing the breakdown of many tissues from age and injury.

The Basics of Cartilage

Your skin, organs, and glands—virtually your entire physical being—consist of a biological matrix woven with threads of proteins, fats, minerals, and vitamins. Cartilage is one of the principal soft structural materials of the body. Your nose, ears, tendons, and ligaments are made of it.

The cartilage forming the pads in your joints, such as your knees and elbows, is denser than other types of cartilage and slightly different in composition from them. These pads are known as "articular cartilage" because they are located where the body articulates, or moves. Articular cartilage in the knees absorbs the impact of walking, thus keeping the interlocking bones of joints from grinding against each other. Similarly, articular cartilage in the elbows, fingers, and mandibular joints of the jaw cushion against impact but also provide a smooth surface that allows joints to swivel and swing. When articular cartilage wears out, the bones themselves rub against one another, leading to excessive wear and tear, inflammation, and pain. Cartilage, in turn, consists largely of collagen, one of the principal proteins of the body.

The best way to think about glucosamine, chondroitin, and vitamin C is as the bricks and mortar of cartilage. Chondroitin typically refers to a group of chemical compounds called glycosaminoglycans, which form cartilage. These compounds are produced by cartilage cells called chondrocytes. Glucosamine stimulates the conversion of glycosaminoglycans to proteoglycans, which give cartilage its resiliency. Vitamin C is involved in some of the chemical reactions that form cartilage. That's about as technical as this chapter will get.

Cartilage breaks down throughout life and is replaced by new cartilage. However, production of new cartilage declines with age, partly because of growing cellular inefficiency and probably because of inadequate nutritional (biochemical) support as well. This is why osteoarthritis is usually but not always age-related. Athletic injuries, particularly to knee joints, accelerate the destruction of articular cartilage and, in effect, speed the aging of joints. Although research shows that glucosamine, chondroitin, and vitamin C supplements help rebuild articular cartilage, bear in mind that they also can help reinforce cartilage throughout the body.

Recent Studies on Glucosamine, Chondroitin, and Vitamin C

Several recent studies, using similar combinations of supplements, clearly convey the benefits of glucosamine, chondroitin, and vitamin C in people with osteoarthritis. In particular, glucosamine and chondroitin help rebuild articular cartilage and also have anti-inflammatory properties, which may explain why they reduce joint pain. These two actions likely reduce the influx of white blood cells into joints, where they would release inflammation-promoting free radicals.

In one study, Alan F. Philippi, M.D., of the U.S. Navy treated thirty-two navy SEALs in their forties who had chronic knee or low-back pain or both. For eight weeks some of the subjects received daily supplements containing 1,500 mg of glucosamine hydrochloride, 1,200 mg of chondroitin sulfate, and 228 mg of manganese ascorbate (a form of vitamin C). Meanwhile, other subjects received placebos, and all the subjects were crossed over to the opposite regimen for another eight weeks.

During the study about half of the patients with osteoarthritis of the knees improved, with reductions of 26 to 43 percent in symptoms, while taking the supplements. However, the supplements did not help with low-back pain.

In a separate clinical trial, Amal K. Das Jr., M.D., of Hendersonville Orthopedics Associates, Hendersonville, N.C., asked ninety-three patients with knee osteoarthritis to take 2,000 mg of glucosamine hydrochloride, 1,600 mg of chondroitin sulfate, and 304 mg of manganese ascorbate or to take placebos daily for six months.

Fifty-two percent of patients with mild or moderate osteoarthritis of the knee benefited from symptom reductions of 25 percent or more after taking the dietary supplements. In contrast, only about half that number of patients improved with the placebo.

Perhaps the most significant recent study was directed by Jean-Yves Reginster, M.D., of the University of Liège, Belgium. He and his fellow Belgian, Italian, and British researchers used digitized X rays to carefully measure the rate of knee cartilage damage in 106 patients with osteoarthritis. The patients then took either 1,500 mg of glucosamine sulfate or a placebo daily for three years.

People taking glucosamine had an average negligible loss of 0.06 millimeter in joint space, and many patients actually gained new cartilage. In contrast, people taking the placebo had a much greater 0.31-millimeter loss in joint space. Reginster reported that people taking glucosamine had a 20 to 25 percent improvement in symptoms, whereas those taking place-bos has a slight worsening. In addition, twice as many patients taking placebos had significant degeneration of their joints compared with those taking glucosamine.

Is It the Glucosamine or the Sulfur That Works?

A recent study by L. John Hoffer, M.D., Ph.D., of Jewish General Hospital, Montréal, suggested that the sulfur (sulfate), not the glucosamine, may be why glucosamine sulfate supplements help rebuild articular cartilage. Sulfur is essential for life, although it is not officially regarded as an essential nutrient. The mineral helps form many of the chemical bonds that hold together skin, collagen, cartilage, and other tissues.

In an article in the journal *Metabolism,* Hoffer pointed out that sulfur is needed for glycosaminoglycan synthesis. However, glucosamine sulfate supplements do not raise blood levels of glucosamine, while they do boost blood sulfur levels. The absorption of sulfur suggests that it is the more biologically active part of the compound, so Hoffer gave 1 gram of glucosamine sulfate to seven healthy subjects; three hours later they had a 13 percent increase in blood sulfur levels. These findings did not directly confirm that glucosamine sulfate helps in osteoarthritis, but they did suggest a biological explanation for why it might work. Also, Hoffer found that when the glucosamine sulfate was given along with acetaminophen (Tylenol), blood sulfur levels dropped by almost 11 percent.

A Controversy: Is Glucosamine Safe in Diabetes?

In 1999 a letter to the journal *Lancet* raised questions about whether glucosamine supplements could increase glucose (blood sugar) levels, cause insulin resistance, and lead to or aggravate diabetes. The questions raised in this letter were widely reported in the *University of California Berkeley Wellness Letter,* the *Tufts University Health & Nutrition Letter,* and other publications toward the end of that year (the delay resulting from publication schedules). These newsletters warned that glucosamine supplements could lead to or worsen diabetes.

But just as those newsletters were being mailed to subscribers, *Lancet* published several letters in response to the original one. Unfortunately, it was too late, and the warnings about glucosamine were starting to become a minor urban (i.e., false) legend, to be repeated by health reporters across the country. Follow-up letters to *Lancet* noted that the original statements were speculative and based only on limited animal research. In contrast, clinical experiences with humans indicated that glucosamine supplements had a tendency to slightly lower blood sugar levels, which would reduce the risk of diabetes. One researcher reported that glucosamine supplements improved wound healing, reduced headaches, and eased inflammatory bowel disease in patients. None of these "side benefits" were reported by the above-named Berkeley and Tufts publications.

Joan: Vitamins and Psoriasis

Since her early twenties, Joan had suffered from psoriasis, which was treated with limited success over the years with a variety of medications. At age fifty-six she visited Richard P. Huemer, M.D., a nutritionally oriented physician in Lancaster, California. Huemer confirmed the original diagnosis of psoriasis, based on characteristic skin lesions, measleslike rashing, and scaling.

He also diagnosed Joan with intestinal dysbiosis, which can result in myriad symptoms, including allergylike symptoms and skin disorders. He recommended that Joan take digestive aid supplements as well as vitamin C, vitamin E, and gamma-linolenic acid supplements. Huemer also recommended homeopathic remedies, including graphites (6X). He also suggested that Joan use Dovonex, a cream containing a form of vitamin D, but Joan did not follow up on this.

Joan's psoriasis improved over the next several months. After four months she was pleased to report to Huemer that her friends told her she no longer had any signs of psoriasis.

Vitamin C and Your Health

Although vitamin C became controversial after Nobel laureate Linus Pauling, Ph.D., recommended supplements to treat the common cold and influenza, the vitamin has many varied and essential roles in maintaining health.

Cartilage and virtually all other tissues in the body are built with large amounts of collagen, a protein often described as the body's "tissue cement." Vitamin C plays an essential role in the synthesis of enzymes needed during the manufacture of collagen. In other words, a complete lack of vitamin C would lead to a disintegration of our skin, organs, and glands. Vitamin C also is needed for the body's synthesis of carnitine, which plays a pivotal role in burning fat for energy, so without vitamin C, we would also feel very fatigued. In addition, vitamin C is one of the major water-soluble antioxidants in the body, protecting against dangerous free radicals.

From a biological standpoint, we may need far more than the 90 mg daily officially recommended for men and women. The rationale for higher levels of vitamin C comes from an examination of vitamin C in other animals. Nearly every mammal—and there are four thousand species—makes its own vitamin C, converting blood sugar to the vitamin. The only exceptions are humans, a handful of higher primates, guinea pigs, and one species of bat. The evolutionary evidence indicates that a common ancestor of humans and some primates lost the ability to make vitamin C about 35 million years ago. Humans still carry the gene that programs for vitamin C production, but it is damaged and nonfunctional.

In the animal kingdom vitamin C is produced at a rate equivalent to 1.8 to 13 grams daily in a person weighing about 150 pounds. The official recommended daily intake for vitamin C ranges from less than 1 percent to 5 percent of this range. One view is that people no longer require as much vitamin C. Another view is that while people lost their ability to make vitamin C, they did not lose their requirement for large amounts of it. One of vitamin C's key roles is in maintaining homeostasis—that is, physiological stability. When stressed, animals increase their production of vitamin C. In humans, stress just seems to exacerbate the vitamin C deficit.

Vitamin C and Inflammatory Disorders

The inability to convert blood sugar to vitamin C may very well predispose people to adult-onset diabetes; excess glucose remains in the blood instead of being converted to vitamin C. Indeed, the chemical similarities between blood sugar and vitamin C lead to a competition between them; both molecules enter the cell on the same transporter protein. This competition takes on greater significance when one considers that diabetes has a strong inflammatory component. People with diabetes typically have elevated levels of interleukin-6 and C-reactive protein. Increasing vitamin C consumption can displace some of the abnormally high blood sugar and improve glucose metabolism.

In particular, vitamin C (like many other antioxidants) appears to dampen inflammation by quenching free radicals and reducing the activity of pro-inflammatory adhesion molecules. Conversely, inadequate intake of vitamin E is associated with inflammatory disorders. For example, a report in the journal *Circulation* noted that patients with peripheral arterial disease (affecting the legs) were more likely to have greater inflammation and severe heart disease when their blood levels of vitamin C were low.

Using Glucosamine, Chondroitin, and Vitamin C

In the past people often obtained the building blocks of cartilage by chewing meat down to the bone, eating gristle attached to meat, or by making soups with bones. Boiling the bones in water releases glucosamine and chondroitin, which are consumed as part of the soup. Research has shown that these substances migrate after digestion to cartilage tissues in people.

The two principal forms of glucosamine in supplements are glucosamine sulfate and glucosamine hydrochloride, and both appear to be equally effective. There is evidence suggesting that glucosamine and chondroitin sulfate are synergistic, with glucosamine enhancing the production of new cartilage and chondroitin slowing the breakdown of cartilage. Many supplements contain both, and people with osteoarthritis should consider taking 1,200 to 1,500 mg of glucosamine and 1,200 mg of chondroitin daily. As part of an osteoarthritic regimen, 500 to 1,000 mg of vitamin C should be included. Although some of the described studies used manganese ascorbate, this type of vitamin C is difficult to find. Any form of vitamin C should suffice.

In general, it would be worthwhile for every person to consume a minimum of 500 mg of supplemental vitamin C. The recent recommendation of 90 mg daily was based on studies of young, healthy men and women. Older people and those with medical conditions very likely will require far more. A far better dosage would be 2,000 to 5,000 mg daily. Robert Cathcart III, M.D., a leading expert in the clinical use of vitamin C to fight infections, developed the "bowel tolerance" method of determining the ideal individual dosage. Using this method, divide your total daily vitamin C dosage into three or four doses over the course of a day, such as with each meal and before bed. Then increase each of the dosages until your stools soften. At that point, reduce your dosage slightly. The dosage will vary from person to person, on average between 1,000 mg and 10,000 mg (10 grams) daily, and your tolerance of vitamin C will increase when you are sick.

In this chapter we have explored the roles of glucosamine, chondroitin, and vitamin C in the body's production of cartilage and collagen, proteins that form a large part of our physical structure. While many nutrients are needed for health, these three nutrients stand out for their roles in reversing osteoarthritis and other inflammatory diseases. In the next chapter you will learn about a variety of other nutrients that also have anti-inflammatory properties.

CHAPTER 11

B Vitamins and More to Reduce Inflammation

In a sense, all essential nutrients play roles in the body's management of inflammation, because all such nutrients help maintain overall health. However, a number of additional nutrients, as well as herbs, stand out for their anti-inflammatory or health-regenerating, properties. These nutrients work in a variety of ways. For example, some B vitamins prevent inflammation-triggering damage to artery walls, whereas some antioxidants inhibit specific inflammation-promoting substances. Herbs also work in a number of ways, as antioxidants and as mild Cox-2 inhibitors.

This chapter describes approximately two dozen additional supplements and herbs that can be of benefit in inflammatory disorders. In general, these supplements should be tried after you have followed the Anti-Inflammation Syndrome Diet Plan and principal inflammation-reversing supplements. Some of these supplements, such as Pycnogenol, have powerful anti-inflammatory effects; it may be worthwhile trying it and others one at a time for one or two months each. The culinary herbs can and should be added as flavorings to meals.

Why not take several of these supplements at once? Doing so may very well alleviate some of your inflammatory symptoms, but you would not know whether you were obtaining the benefits from one or most or all of the supplements you decided to take. You might say that that doesn't matter if you feel better quickly, but it could be a more costly approach than identifying the individual supplement or supplements that help you the most. Finally, it is worth pointing out that you probably would not want or need to consume all of the following nutrients, for financial reasons if nothing else.

Dorothy: Nutritional Supplements to Treat Cancer

Abram Hoffer, M.D., Ph.D., one of the pioneers in vitamin therapy, initially began treating cancer patients for depression and anxiety. He soon found that patients taking large dosages of vitamin C and other vitamins and minerals were living longer than those who did not. When his cases were analyzed by Nobel laureate Linus Pauling, Ph.D., it became clear that cancer patients were living several times longer (postdiagnosis) when they took supplements, compared with patients who chose not to take supplements.

Hoffer has treated more than twelve hundred cancer patients since 1977, and some types of cancer (such as breast and prostate) are more responsive to supplements than other types (such as lung). One of his patients is Dorothy of Victoria, British Columbia, Canada.

Dorothy was first diagnosed with breast cancer in 1975, when she was forty-nine years old and going through an emotionally draining divorce. Doctors performed a lumpectomy, gave her radiation therapy, and pronounced her treated and cured.

But conventional medicine didn't cure Dorothy. Her cancer eventually reappeared in one of her breasts and also spread to her lungs. For the past few years, however, she has been healthy and free of cancer. Dorothy credits her long-term survival to "quality" vitamin supplements, a good diet, and a great attitude toward life.

For many years Dorothy took large amounts of vitamin A to reduce the risk of metastasis. However, the cancer did metastasize to her lungs in 1995, but it receded after drug treatment.

In 1997 she consulted with Hoffer, and she has since been taking a high-powered assortment of nutritional supplements, including vitamins A, C, D, and E, beta-carotene, selenium, and the vitaminlike coenzyme Q_{10}. "I do feel I need these extra supplements," Dorothy says. "I think anyone in this situation would need them."

Dorothy emphasizes organic foods in her diet, eating a lot of fish, vegetables, and occasionally game meats (deer, elk). In her midseventies, Dorothy is physically active—much more so than many other seniors who have not battled cancer. She soothes her soul and reduces stress with music, meditation, visualization, long walks, and a positive mental attitude.

The B-Complex Vitamins

Several B vitamins, including folic acid and vitamins B_6 and B_{12}, can lower blood levels of homocysteine, a toxic amino acid that damages blood vessel walls, initiates localized inflammation, and increases the risk of coronary artery disease and stroke.

Homocysteine plays a role in normal biochemistry. It is formed as a by-product of methionine, an essential amino acid found in protein. However, homocysteine should exist relatively briefly in the related chemical reactions, and blood levels should remain low. Folic acid and vitamin B_{12} help convert homocysteine back to methionine, and vitamin B_6 helps convert to cystathionine, another necessary compound in the reactions.

However, when a person has low levels of one or more of these vitamins, homocysteine cannot be converted, and blood levels rise. This imbalance usually occurs for one of several reasons: too much protein, too few B vitamins, or a common genetic defect that partially interferes with how the body uses folic acid. Without sufficient B vitamins, homocysteine injures blood vessel walls, particularly those in the heart and brain. This injury triggers an immune response, attracting white blood cells to the blood vessel wall and damaging it.

It is best to maintain homocysteine levels as low as possible—4 to 6 micromoles (mmoles) per liter of blood is ideal. The risk of heart disease noticeably increases when levels increase. A level of 10 mmoles is abnormally elevated, and 13 or higher is very dangerous. Folic acid supplements by themselves can generally lower homocysteine levels, and health food stores sell several brands of homocysteine-lowering supplements, which generally contain two other B vitamins. However, it might be better to simply take a high-potency B-complex supplement. Look for a B-complex supplement containing 10 to 25 mg of vitamin B_1—this is a clue to the higher potency of other B vitamins in the formula.

The B vitamins exert an analgesic effect as well. A paper published in the German medical journal *Schmerz* (which means "pain") described how vitamins B_1, B_6, and B_{12}, especially when taken in combination, reduce musculoskeletal pain and enhance the effects of nonsteroidal anti-inflammatory drugs (NSAIDs). A separate study, which focused on 303 elderly American veterans, found body pain strongly associated with a deficiency of vitamin B_{12}, which affected more than one-fifth of the subjects.

Flavonoids and Polyphenols

As a family of vitaminlike nutrients, flavonoids and polyphenols possess striking anti-inflammatory properties. More than five thousand flavonoids, sometimes referred to as bioflavonoids, have been identified in plants, and they are part of a larger group of water-soluble chemical antioxidants known as polyphenols. All of these compounds function as light-absorbing plant pigments; as they absorb light, they limit the formation of hazardous free radicals. Flavonoids and polyphenols provide the blue in blueberries and the red in raspberries and strawberries. (Some of the other colors are the result of carotenoids. See "Beta-Carotene" on page 143.) It is likely that in a diet that includes a variety of fresh fruits and vegetables, a person consumes hundreds if not thousands of these antioxidants.

Flavonoids and polyphenols provide the lion's share of antioxidants in fruits and vegetables. For example, 100 g (about 3.5 oz) of a fresh apple provides about 5.7 mg of vitamin C. However, the same apple, including the skin, contains 219 mg of flavonoids and 290 mg of other polyphenols, which together are equivalent to the antioxidant activity of about 1,500 mg of vitamin C. Eating a variety of fruits and vegetables likely provides several hundred different types of flavonoids and/or polyphenols. All of these flavonoids and polyphenols are related and often form new compounds, creating a chemical kaleidoscope of antioxidants. All of these different chemical structures are like thousands of puzzle pieces, matching up to the many different types of inflammation-promoting free radicals.

Quercetin

One of the most popular flavonoid supplements is also one of the most misunderstood. Quercetin (pronounced kwair-sih-tin), found in apples and onions, can inhibit the activity of some types of adhesion molecules, which promote many types of inflammatory reactions. Adhesion molecules enable white blood cells, which secrete pro-inflammatory compounds, to attach to normal cells. In terms of chemical structure, quercetin is similar to both rutin, another naturally occurring flavonoid, and to cromolyn sodium (NasalCrom), a synthetic flavonoid drug used to prevent pollen allergies.

Many physicians have found quercetin supplements, 300 to 500 mg daily, helpful in treating pollen allergies, but there is a catch. Quercetin supplements have failed to pass the Ames test for mutagenicity, which means they cause breaks in genetic material and conceivably could increase the risk of cancer. In practical terms this risk may be remote because fruits and vegetables supply many nutrients that enhance the body's repair mechanisms. But still, there is something troubling about taking a potential carcinogen to treat inflammation or allergies. Only one form of quercetin has passed the Ames test. That is quercetin chalcone, made by Thorne Research (208-263-1337).

Pycnogenol and Grape Seed Extract

Pycnogenol (pronounced pick-noj'-in-nall) is a patented complex of about forty antioxidants, mostly proanthocyanidins (a family of flavonoids) and a variety of other antioxidants, including organic acids (such as cinnamic acids, caffeic acid, and ferulic acid). It is extracted from the bark of French maritime pine trees and sold under the Pycnogenol brand name by many different companies.

The many different antioxidants in Pycnogenol make its sum far greater than any of its individual parts. Studies by Lester Packer, Ph.D., an antioxidant expert and professor emeritus at the University of California, Berkeley, have found that Pycnogenol is a powerful antioxidant. In addition to quenching free radicals, it also turns off some of the genes involved in producing inflammation. One study has found that Pycnogenol supplements reduced inflammation in patients with lupus erythematosus.

Traditionally, Pycnogenol is best known for strengthening blood vessel walls, preventing the leakage of blood and abnormal bruising. It is likely that it achieves these benefits partly by inhibiting inflammation in blood vessel walls. Studies with laboratory animals have determined that it is a powerful anti-inflammatory nutrient. In addition, many physicians have found that Pycnogenol supplements, ranging from 25 to 200 mg daily, can often have dramatic effects in people with rheumatic diseases.

Pycnogenol works in part by inhibiting production of peroxides, which stimulate inflammatory activity in white blood cells. In a laboratory experiment, researchers found that Pycnogenol reduced peroxide formation and increased levels of glutathione, an anti-inflammatory antioxidant.

Grape seed extracts are also rich in proanthocyanidins, though the specific types of antioxidants in this supplement are somewhat different from those in Pycnogenol. Grape seed extracts have a similar effect on blood vessel walls, and they also possess anti-inflammatory properties. Some of the physicians who use both supplements feel that there are subtle differences between the two in patient responses. It may be worthwhile to try one, then the other to see if one is better for you.

Glutathione Boosters

Glutathione is the principal antioxidant made by the body, though it is commonly found in foods with other antioxidants. Glutathione supplements are generally unreliable because the molecule may be broken down during digestion. Taking almost any antioxidant supplement, such as vitamin E or vitamin C, will increase the body's production of glutathione. The following three supplements are particularly good glutathione boosters because they contain precursors of glutathione.

N-acetylcysteine

N-acetylcysteine (NAC) is an exceptionally safe form of the amino acid cysteine. Its safety is important to note because pure cysteine can become neurotoxic at high dosages. Cysteine is a direct precursor to glutathione and the many different glutathione compounds made and used in the body.

NAC is used in every hospital emergency room in the nation to treat overdoses of acetaminophen (Tylenol). Acetaminophen depletes liver levels of glutathione and, in large amounts, can rapidly lead to liver failure. NAC quickly rebuilds normal glutathione levels in the liver, which then helps the organ break down and detoxify the drug. The same glutathione-enhancing effect of NAC has also been found to increase the life expectancy of people with AIDS, which depletes glutathione levels.

The National Cancer Institute has studied NAC as a potential cancer-preventive nutrient, but the most dramatic study published was actually on NAC and flu symptoms. Silvio De Flora, M.D., of the University of Genoa, Italy, gave 262 elderly subjects either 1,200 mg of NAC or placebos daily during the winter flu season. Although NAC did not prevent flu infections, it had a "striking" effect on symptoms. Of the subjects with laboratory-confirmed flus, only 25 percent of those taking NAC developed flu symptoms, and they were generally mild and of short duration. In contrast, 79 percent of the people taking placebos had more severe flu symptoms, according to De Flora's article in the *European Respiratory*

Journal. This symptom-reducing effect is very important in controlling inflammation related to infection.

Alpha-Lipoic Acid

This antioxidant, found in spinach and beef, is approved in Germany for the treatment of diabetic neuropathy (nerve disease). Several studies have found that it can greatly improve insulin function and reduce blood sugar levels by 10 to 30 percent in diabetics. Like NAC, alpha-lipoic acid is a sulfur-containing molecule that may be a more efficient glutathione booster.

Research over the past twenty-five years by Burton M. Berkson, M.D., Ph.D., an adjunct professor at New Mexico State University, Las Cruces, has found alpha-lipoic acid to greatly enhance liver function and liver glutathione levels. This effect is particularly important in controlling chronic hepatitis. Patients with hepatitis C consistently and significantly improve when following his "triple antioxidant" regimen, which included 600 mg of alpha-lipoic acid, 400 mcg of selenium, and 900 mg of silymarin (an extract of the herb milk thistle) daily. This program leads to a near normalization of liver function.

Selenium

Selenium is an essential dietary mineral and an essential part of several glutathione peroxidases, powerful antioxidant and anti-inflammatory enzymes made by the body. Selenium supplements, 200 mcg daily, increase the body's production of glutathione peroxidases. These compounds enhance resistance to infection, which reduces one source of inflammatory reactions and also prevents very dangerous mutations in flu and other viruses. In addition, a human trial at the University of Arizona, Tucson, found that selenium supplements reduced the risk of breast and prostate cancers by about half.

Cynthia: Antioxidants to Treat Hepatitis

At age thirty-three, Cynthia had received a blood transfusion following the birth of her daughter. Several weeks later she developed a general sense of fatigue, along with muscle pains and jaundice. She quickly became too sick to care for her daughter.

Laboratory tests indicated that Cynthia had contracted hepatitis C, and her physician noted that the virus also had damaged her pancreas, resulting in elevated blood sugar levels and diabetes. Her prognosis was poor, but a specialist suggested that she have an injection of interferon and an antiviral drug, which would result in flulike symptoms for about six months. In addition, Cynthia was told that she would eventually need a liver transplant.

Seeking an alternative to interferon therapy and a liver transplant, Cynthia consulted with Burton M. Berkson, M.D., Ph.D., of Las Cruces, New Mexico. At the time she was fatigued and her liver was enlarged and tender. Tests indicated that her liver enzymes were very high and her fasting blood sugar level was 300 mg/dl. (Normal is 75 to 85 mg/dl.)

Berkson started Cynthia on his "triple antioxidant" approach, which included 600 mg of alpha-lipoic acid, 400 mcg of selenium, and 900 mg of silymarin daily. He also asked her to follow a diet similar to the Anti-Inflammation Syndrome Diet Plan, rich in protein and vegetables and low in refined carbohydrates. After two weeks she had an increase in energy and was able to resume many normal activities. By the sixth week of supplementation Cynthia's liver enzymes had fallen to near-normal levels and her fasting glucose was 112 mg/dl. She has been following the diet and supplement regimen for more than five years and reports that she still feels great.

Beta-Carotene

In addition to flavonoids, fruits and vegetables contain large quantities of carotenoids, a family of fat-soluble antioxidants. Several studies suggest that these nutrients—chiefly beta-carotene, lutein, and lycopene—are associated with relatively low levels of C-reactive protein (CRP). This association does not necessarily mean that carotenoids lower CRP levels, though this effect would be consistent with other research on antioxidants. Carotenoid levels might simply reflect fruit and vegetable consumption and the combined anti-inflammatory action of carotenoids, flavonoids, and vitamins.

In one study of several thousand people, researchers found that high levels of all the major dietary carotenoids were associated with low levels of inflammatory markers, including CRP. Another group of researchers found that both CRP and high white blood cell counts, another marker or inflammation, were associated with low beta-carotene levels. All of the major dietary carotenoids neutralize peroxinitrite, a type of free radical that increases inflammation.

Methylsulfonylmethane (MSM)

This supplement consists of about one-third elemental sulfur, a nutrient that exists in nutritional limbo. Sulfur is not considered an essential nutrient, but every indication points to its crucial role in health and life itself. Glutathione, NAC, and alpha-lipoic acid all contain sulfur molecules. So does the B vitamin biotin, the anticoagulant heparin, and the hormone insulin. Sulfur also is an integral part of the biological cement that forms skin, hair, nails, and the cartilage that shapes your nose and pads your joints.

Published, controlled studies on MSM are limited, but more than fifty-five thousand studies have been published on a very similar molecule, dimethyl sulfoxide (DMSO). Stanley Jacob, M.D., of Oregon Health Sciences University, Portland, a pioneer in researching both substances, has found MSM very effective in reducing muscle and joint pain, interstitial cystitis (a type of very painful bladder inflammation), and even pollen allergies in some people.

Dietitians have generally assumed that people obtain sufficient sulfur through dietary methionine and cysteine. However, the extraordinary successes obtained by Jacob suggest that other chemical forms of sulfur (besides those in amino acids) may be readily used in the body. Jacob recommends daily supplementation of 1,000 to 2,000 mg daily, though larger amounts are safe.

S-adenosyl-L-methionine

Usually referred to as SAMe (pronounced "sammy"), this sulfur-containing nutrient donates "methyl groups" to more than forty major chemical reactions in the body. Methyl groups provide carbon and hydrogen and are necessary for creating new cells. SAMe has often been recommended for treating inflammation and arthritis: it donates sulfur molecules to glucosamine and chondroitin sulfate, enabling the body to build new collagen and cartilage.

SAMe also has been found helpful in treating depression, though B-complex vitamins can boost SAMe levels and are less expensive. Its benefit in depression suggests a common biochemical defect with inflammation. Depression is frequently associated with some inflammatory diseases such as asthma, Alzheimer's, coronary artery disease, and diabetes.

Herbs and Spices

Medicinal and culinary herbs are rich sources of anti-inflammatory antioxidants, especially flavonoids. They also contain trace amounts of natural Cox-2 inhibitors, such as salicylates. Medicinal herbs can be especially potent, while culinary herbs are perhaps less potent but more tasty anti-inflammatory nutrients.

Over the past several years herbal medicines have moved from folk-medicine status to scientifically supported treatments. Major drug companies routinely fund expeditions to the Amazon and other undeveloped regions to identify new plants and potentially therapeutic molecules. Almost half of all modern drugs have either been developed from plant compounds or are synthetic replicas of molecules found in plants.

Unlike pharmaceutical drugs, which are usually built around a single synthetic molecule, herbs may contain hundreds if not thousands of active principles. The diversity and frequent synergism of these anti-inflammatory compounds lead to a multifaceted biochemical attack on inflammation, instead of overwhelming a single biochemical pathway and causing side effects. In fact, many of the substances in herbs are also found in common fruits and vegetables, which means they have historically played a role in human nutrition and evolution. Indeed, the anti-inflammatory nutrients in fruits, vegetables, and herbs may have historically helped control excessive inflammation.

Devil's Claw

Devil's claw *(Harpagophytum procumbens)* is a traditional southern African herb used to treat pain and upset stomachs. Its name comes from its clawlike fruit, which resemble the feet of birds. Ten clinical studies conducted between 1982 and 2000 have found that devil's claw can benefit people with rheumatoid arthritis, low back pain, and various other rheumatic complaints.

In the June 2000 issue of *Phytomedicine,* French researchers reported using devil's claw to successfully treat ninety-two people with osteoarthritis. The subjects were given either 435 mg of powdered devil's claw or conventional drug treatment daily. By the end of the four-month studies, people taking devil's claw had significantly less pain and greater mobility. They were also relying on fewer anti-inflammatory drugs and painkillers. Similar results were noted in a broader study, which included 122 patients with either hip or knee osteoarthritis or both.

Cat's Claw

Despite a similar name, cat's claw *(Uncaria tomentosa)* is unrelated to devil's claw. Cat's claw is native to South America and known as *una de gato* in Peru. Its use as an anti-inflammatory herb dates back hundreds of years, to the Inca civilization.

A recent series of experiments detailed the anti-inflammatory properties of cat's claw. Manuel Sandoval-Chacon, Ph.D., and Mark J. S. Miller, Ph.D., of Albany Medical College, New York, conducted cell and animal experiments to investigate the herb's specific biological properties. In one of the experiments, human cells were exposed to peroxynitrite, a powerful free radical that can destroy cells. When the cells also were exposed to cat's claw, they were protected from the peroxynitrite radicals.

Peroxynitrite also increases levels of pro-inflammatory prostaglandin E_2, and cat's claw would theoretically lower its levels. According to Sandoval-Chacon and Miller, cat's claw also inhibits the activity of NF-kappa B, a protein that turns on inflammation-causing genes. Such findings, the researchers noted, are consistent with the herb's traditional uses. Effective dosages range from 250 to 1,000 mg of cat's claw extract daily.

Chamomile

Chamomile (*Matricaria* species) was used as an herbal remedy by the ancient Egyptians and Romans, and the herb's mild-flavored tea has been recommended for menstrual cramps, stomach pain, indigestion, and fever. The tea, made with a tiny bit of honey, is excellent for treating an upset stomach. Used topically, chamomile poultices, lotions, and creams can have cosmetic and dermatologic benefits as well.

In Germany, which makes extensive use of pharmaceutical-grade herbs, chamomile is regarded as the first choice for treating mild skin problems, such as rashes, in infants. A human study of nine healthy women found that topically applied chamomile was absorbed deeply into the skin. Not surprisingly, then, many cosmetics (such as the Camo-Care brand) use chamomile.

The active components of chamomile include blue azulene (an essential oil), glycosides (carbohydrate-based compounds found in many medicinal plants), and many acids and esters. It is also rich in antioxidants. In an unpublished study allergist Holger Biltz, M.D., of Bad Honnef, Germany, reported that a chamomile-containing cream reduced reddening after UV exposure, and reduced skin roughness.

Green Tea

Green tea and, to a lesser extent, black tea are rich sources of antioxidant flavonoids known as catechins. These catechins include three closely related antioxidants: epigallocatechin-3 gallate (EGCG), epigallocatechin (EGC), and epicatechin-3 gallate (ECG). Together they form about 30 percent of the dry weight of tea leaves. The sheer quantity of catechins in green tea point to their remarkable antioxidant power.

Dozens of studies by Japanese researchers—avid drinkers of green tea—have shown that catechins can prevent free-radical damage to cholesterol and lower the risk of heart disease and cancer. Population-based studies have shown that tea drinkers have a lower than average risk of heart disease, stroke, and several cancers, including esophageal, stomach, and lung cancers.

The protective properties of green tea can be traced, at least in part, to the anti-inflammatory properties of catechins. These substances can inhibit the formation of pro-inflammatory compounds, and they have mild analgesic effects as well. In one study Japanese researchers reported that EGCG could inhibit the release of histamine, the compound that causes the itchy feeling in allergies.

A separate study, conducted at Case Western Reserve University, Cleveland, Ohio, tested the effects of green tea in arthritic laboratory mice. Only about half of the mice drinking green tea developed a serious form of arthritis, and the other animals in the green-tea group had only a mild form of the disease. In contrast, all but one of the mice drinking only water developed arthritis. In other words, green tea (in amounts comparable to what a person might drink) significantly reduced the likelihood of developing and the severity of arthritis in mice.

Bromelain

Bromelain is an enzyme found in pineapple stems, and it has been widely used to treat athletic injuries. It seems to reduce the sense of pain and heat in inflammation, and it may be of use in other conditions, such as colitis and arthritis.

This enzyme has some anticlotting properties, which may be why it has sometimes been recommended in the treatment of coronary artery disease. In fact, some pro-inflammatory eicosanoids (by-products of omega-6 fatty acids) promote clotting, whereas anti-inflammatory eicosanoids (by-products of omega-3 fatty acids) reduce blood clotting. Bromelain is best taken on an empty stomach, and 600 mg daily are worth trying for inflammation.

Boswellia

Boswellia is the common name for the resins of *Boswellia serrata,* a tree that grows in India. These resins have been used in traditional Ayurvedic medicine, and they are rich in a group of anti-inflammatory compounds described as boswellic acids.

Boswellia inhibits 5-lipoxygenase, one of the enzymes needed for the body's production of inflammatory compounds. It also seems to break some of the links in the inflammatory chain reaction involving what physicians know as "complement." While complement is an essential part of our immune defenses, its overactivity can contribute to chronic inflammation.

Several studies have used 200 mg of boswellic acid extracts three times daily to treat rheumatoid arthritis, osteoarthritis, and associated inflammation. These studies have shown a reduction in symptoms, such as pain and morning stiffness, as well as in inflammatory markers. Preliminary research also suggests that these extracts may ease asthma as well.

Feverfew

The herb feverfew *(Tanacetum parthenium)* was used in ancient Greece to treat headaches and, as the name indicates, fevers. It is currently approved as an over-the-counter product in Canada for the specific treatment of migraine headaches. Like other herbs, it is sold in the United States and other countries without a specific therapeutic claim.

Its active ingredient, parthenolide, stabilizes blood vessel tension. Although it is of limited use during an actual migraine headache, the herb's long-term use does reduce the frequency of migraine headaches. Dosages of feverfew products vary among brands, but one of the most reliable brands (available at health food stores) is MygraFew, made by Nature's Way.

In 2001 researchers at Yale University (New Haven, Connecticut) determined that parthenolide had potentially far-reaching anti-inflammatory properties. They identified the molecular basis of the herb, showing that it disrupts the function of "IkappaB kinase beta," an inflammation-triggering compound.

Elder

Elder leaves and elderberries (*Sambucus nigra* and other species) have a long history of medicinal use. Hippocrates, regarded as the father of medicine, wrote about elderberries in the fourth century B.C. Shakespeare mentioned them in his play *The Merry Wives of Windsor.* They were viewed as so potent that during the 1600s, many people hung elderberry branches and leaves by their doors to keep away the evil spirits that were believed to cause illness. Among Native Americans, various species of elder leaves were used to treat rheumatism and fever.

Laboratory experiments have confirmed the anti-inflammatory properties of elder leaves. Leaf extracts reduce levels of several pro-inflammation cytokines. Meanwhile, a syrup made from elderberries was reported, in a double-blind study, to significantly reduce flu symptoms. In the study 90 percent of people taking the elderberry syrup (Sambucol) reported a "complete cure" of their flu symptoms in two to three days, compared with six days for most of the people taking a placebo.

Garlic

Many of the health benefits of garlic *(Allium sativum)* result from its anti-inflammatory properties. For example, garlic is well known as a mild blood thinner. It works by turning down the activity of thromboxanes, which promote blood clotting. The same thromboxanes are also involved in inflammation. Some studies also have found that garlic supplements can lower blood sugar and cholesterol levels, though not all people seem to benefit equally.

Because it is rich in sulfur, garlic also can boost the body's production of glutathione. This food and condiment is a good example of some of the health benefits of oxidation. The chemical constituents of garlic are relatively inert until it is sliced, diced, cooked, or chewed. Breaking up a garlic clove begins a cascade of oxidation reactions (with oxygen), lead-ing to the production of compounds very similar to sulfur-containing amino acids. All forms of garlic—supplements, powders, and fresh—ap-pear to have benefits, though supplements and freshly prepared appear to be the most potent.

It makes sense to use ample garlic in your meals. Its adds tremendous flavor, even if it had no health benefits. Garlic supplements concentrate levels of some of the active constituents, but their advertising can be con-fusing. The major brands are Kwai, Kyolic, Pure-Gar, and Garlicin. Be-cause each product is produced differently, each contains a slightly different group of compounds. Dosages of 500 to 1,000 mg daily may have an anti-inflammatory effect.

Ginger

Few spices besides gingerroot are versatile enough to flavor both entrées and desserts, from Oriental meals to gingerbread cookies. Native to South Asia, ginger *(Zingiber officinale)* has become a popular spice around the world.

Gingerroot has well-documented anti-inflammatory properties. It is rich in kaempferol, a flavonoid that functions in part as a mild Cox-2 inhibitor. In addition, ginger blocks lipoxygenase, another enzyme involved in the body's production of inflammatory compounds. Ginger also appears to contain trace amounts of melatonin, a hormone other-wise made by the pineal gland; melatonin has antioxidant and anti-inflammatory properties. (Pure melatonin has sleep-inducing properties, so it is not recommended as an anti-inflammatory supplement.)

Both ginger and ginger-containing supplements have been found helpful in osteoarthritis, rheumatism, and muscular pain. Ginger has the added benefit of reducing nausea. Although ginger is common in grocery stores, the best form (and most difficult to find) is fresh baby gingerroot, which is especially tender.

Curcumin and Turmeric Root

Curcumin, a bright yellow spice, is obtained from the root of turmeric *(Curcuma longa),* a member of the ginger family. Native to Asia, cur-cumin is one of the oldest and most cherished anti-inflammatory herbs in Indian Ayurvedic medicine.

Turmeric root and curcumin are mild Cox-2 inhibitors but are not as powerful and not as dangerous as popular Cox-2-inhibiting drugs. According to recent experiments, they block the activity of "NF kappa B," a protein that turns on inflammation-promoting genes. This effect and similar ones too complex to discuss here also suggest that the herbs also might reduce the risk of cancer. Animal studies have found that turmeric root and curcumin may reduce arthritic symptoms.

Plantain

The herb plantain *(Plantago lanceolata, P. major)* is used in Germany to treat upper respiratory inflammation and to reduce skin inflammation. It is an ingredient in some anticough and expectorant medicines.

One of its chemical components, ursolic acid, it a potent anti-inflammatory. In a study conducted at Uppsala University, Sweden, researchers reported that it was a highly selective inhibitor of Cox-2, the cyclooxygenase enzyme more involved in inflammatory reactions.

Oregano

This common culinary herb may be one of the overlooked reasons why the traditional Greek and Mediterranean diet is associated with a lower risk of heart disease. Oregano *(Origanum vulgare),* a member of the mint family, contains a large number of anti-inflammatory flavonoids and polyphenols, including rosmarinic acid, kaempferol, ursolic acid, and apigenin.

Widely used in Greek and Italian cooking, oregano adds a wonderful flavor to foods. Greek oregano has a stronger smell and flavor than Mexican oregano. Dried oregano is fine as a culinary herb, but it is best when freshly dried.

In this chapter we have explored a variety of vitamins, vitaminlike nutrients, and herbs that have documented anti-inflammatory and healing properties. These nutrients and herbs should be added to the core Anti-Inflammation Syndrome Diet Plan and supplement recommendations, but obviously you cannot take or use all of them all the time. In the next section we will focus on preventing and reversing some of the most common inflammatory disorders.

PART IV

Putting Anti-Inflammation Syndrome Nutrients to Work for You

CHAPTER 12

The Inflammation Syndrome, Diseases, and Specific Conditions

Up to this point we have focused on the leading dietary causes and solutions for the Inflammation Syndrome. In this chapter we shift to specific diseases and conditions that are caused or exacerbated by inflammation—and remedied by improvements in diet and anti-inflammatory supplements.

Inflammatory disorders frequently follow a progression, beginning with mild symptoms that, if the underlying causes remain uncorrected, progress to more serious and difficult-to-treat diseases. For example, gastritis can lead to stomach ulcers and increase the risk of stomach cancer. Similarly, athletic injuries can set the stage for osteoarthritis and chronic musculoskeletal pain. Although symptoms may seem to be mild or transitory during the early stages of an inflammatory disease, it is easier to heal them at this time. In contrast, it is more difficult to reverse established diseases because of the extent of tissue damage.

In addition, inflammatory disorders often occur in clusters, one disorder being linked to another, and often forming the Inflammation Syndrome. These clusters point to similar underlying causes, though the common causes may be overlooked. For example, periodontitis increases the risk of heart disease, making some physicians believe that both diseases have a common infectious cause. Rather, people with the two conditions more likely share a common inflammatory pattern resulting from a pro-inflammatory diet and inadequate intake of vitamins E and C. As another example, people with asthma frequently suffer from depression. The depression does not result from the unfortunate diagnosis of asthma but, instead, may be symptomatic of the same fatty acid imbalance affecting body and mind.

You might wonder why, if most people are eating essentially the same pro-inflammatory diet, one person develops a particular set of symptoms, such as rheumatoid arthritis, whereas another suffers asthmatic attacks, and yet another person has heart disease. The diseases to which you are susceptible reflect your individual biological weaknesses, which are the result of your genetics, overall lifestyle, stresses, age, and diet. To understand this, it helps to see your genes and biochemistry as a series of chainlike links. Everyone has their own set of weak links (as well as strong links), and the number of weak links increases with age, poor diet, stress, and other insults. Your major weak links may be your heart, your joints, or your stomach or some other tissue. Good nutrition reinforces these links and may be more important to health than genetics; this has been borne out by recent research. As you read early in this book, genes themselves depend on adequate levels of nutrients for optimal functioning.

In general, the following sections place more emphasis on conditions affecting larger numbers of people and less emphasis on those affecting fewer people. It would be impossible to cover the full spectrum of inflammatory diseases in this type of book. Still, the Anti-Inflammation Syndrome Diet Plan should have a positive impact on virtually all inflammatory diseases. So if you suffer from a disorder that is not described here, it would be worthwhile trying the diet plan and some of the supplements.

Age-Related Wear and Tear

What Is Age-Related Wear and Tear?

Throughout life, old or damaged cells are broken down and replaced. However, after about age twenty-seven, the rate of cell damage begins to outpace the body's natural repair processes. With poor nutrition, this shift toward greater cellular breakdown may begin at an earlier age. Old cells are not as efficient as new ones, and the accumulation of old cells is what is recognized as aging.

Causes

Wear and tear is a normal part of living and aging. Much of it results from damage by free radicals, according to Denham Harman, M.D., Ph.D., professor emeritus at the University of Nebraska, Omaha. In the 1950s Harman proposed the free-radical theory of aging—that these hazardous molecules chip away at the deoxyribonucleic acid (DNA), proteins, and fats in cells. The cumulative effect is less efficient cell performance and decreased activity of organs, reflected in a weaker heart and weaker lungs, as but two examples. Sometimes free-radical mutations of DNA lead to vastly different cell behavior, such as that of cancer cells.

Most of these free radicals are generated by normal metabolic processes in the body, such as the burning of glucose for energy or the detoxification of dangerous chemicals, such as cigarette smoke. Normally, most of these free radicals are contained in specific chemical reactions, but some do leak out—and additional free radicals may be formed when a person consumes inadequate levels of antioxidants.

Some people seem to age faster than others, a process strongly linked to excessive levels of free radicals. A good example is a woman who maintains a beautiful tan in her twenties and thirties, either by sunning herself on the beach or by using tanning booths. By the time she turns fifty, she will likely have far more facial wrinkles and tougher skin than a person who has minimized exposure to the sun. That's because tanning increases exposure to ultraviolet radiation, which creates free radicals and speeds the aging of skin cells. Athletic injuries also can accelerate the aging process, particularly of joints and bones, and injuries have been documented to create free radicals. The chemicals in cigarette smoke are dangerous in part because they stress the body's ability to detoxify them, generating still more free radicals in the process.

In addition, poor nutrition and leading a hard life increase wear and tear. For example, malnourished people often look ten to fifteen years older than their chronological age. Good nutrition should provide compounds that maintain a normal aging process or, ideally, even slow it down. Inadequate nutrition hurts our natural defenses against a variety of stresses, such as UV radiation, air pollution, and noxious chemicals.

How Common Is Age-Related Wear and Tear?

The sad fact is that everyone ages, and everyone will experience some degree of age-related wear and tear, even while remaining in "good health" late in life. Frailty late in life is one sign of wear and tear.

The Inflammation Syndrome Connection

Much of the cleanup of old cells is performed by the immune system, chiefly various types of white blood cells. Increased wear and tear activates more white blood cells, which are a double-edged sword because they secrete more inflammation-producing chemicals. Immune cells may target specific sites in the body, such as joints, the heart, or bronchi, or migrate and cause more systemic inflammation. A study in the November 11, 2002, *Archives of Internal Medicine* described a strong relationship between frailty in elderly men and women and high levels of C-reactive protein and other signs of chronic inflammation. In addition, frail elderly people also had elevated prediabetic levels of glucose and insulin. All of these factors contribute to the breakdown and aging of tissues—that is, age-related wear and tear—which evolves into a wasting syndrome among many elderly people. Disturbingly, the researchers noted that the 4,700 seniors in their study were healthier on average than most other people in the same age group.

Standard Treatment

There is really no treatment for the normal process of aging, though some hormones may restore many aspects of youthfulness, such as muscle and sexual vigor. Some medications also may improve cognitive function, but nearly all drugs possess undesirable side effects. For example, many hormones can increase cancer risk.

Nutrients That Can Help

Antioxidants such as vitamins E, C, and others often have been described as "antiaging" nutrients because they quench many of the excess free radicals. Consuming a lot of vegetables and fruits and taking antioxidant supplements strengthen the body's defenses against free radicals. Antioxidants also have potent anti-inflammatory properties.

What Else Might Help?

High levels of two hormones, insulin and cortisol, appear to speed the aging process. Insulin is usually regarded as the hormone needed to burn blood sugar, but it is actually a primary anabolic hormone that can increase either muscle or fat. Elevated insulin levels seem to speed the aging process and increase the risk of coronary artery disease. A diet relatively low in refined sugars and carbohydrates, such as the diet described in this book, can help lower blood sugar and insulin levels, which in turn lower inflammation levels.

Cortisol is one of the body's primary stress-response hormones, and high levels stress the body itself, leading to wear and tear. Cortisol also increases the risk of heart attack. The body cannot maintain a biological red alert without paying the price. Stress-reduction techniques as well as the B-complex vitamins can lower cortisol levels.

Allergies, Food

What Are Food Allergies?

Various types of food allergies or food sensitivities (characterized by symptoms, but not confirmed by laboratory tests) can maintain the body's inflammatory response at a high idle. These allergies can exacerbate symptoms of other inflammatory diseases, such as asthma and rheumatoid arthritis, or raise blood pressure and blood sugar levels. Occasionally they can completely mimic the symptoms of other diseases.

Causes

There are several leading causes of food allergies, and they may intertwine. Physicians have traditionally recognized only acute allergic reactions, such as when a person develops a rash after eating shellfish or strawberries. However, most cases of food allergies may be more subtle and difficult to diagnose.

Food Addictions

As ironic as it might seem, some people actually become addicted to a food that causes an allergic reaction. This allergy/addiction may develop as part of the body's response to a commonly consumed allergen. During these reactions, the body releases endorphins, substances that create a natural "high." Any substance that creates a temporary sense of euphoria can become addictive, and in this case people can develop an addiction to the allergenic food, initiating the high.

Often, eating a lot of any particular food (even healthy foods) can create an allergy to it because, inexplicably, it triggers an immune response or it stresses specific digestive enzymes. It is as if too much of any single type of food overloads the body's ability to continue to break it down in the gut. Furthermore, any food can be the source of an allergy/addiction, whether it is junk food or a healthy food. One clue to an allergy/addiction is a food that a person craves. Foods containing chocolate, dairy, wheat, corn, tomatoes, and soy are among the most common food allergens.

Celiac Disease

Wheat, rye, barley, and most (but not all) grains contain gluten, a term used to describe a family of about forty proteins. People who are gluten-sensitive often develop celiac disease, but nonceliac gluten sensitivity may be common. The immune response to gluten can damage the wall of the intestine, resulting in explosive bowel movements, poor nutrient absorption, and a consequential increased risk of dozens of diseases. Celiac disease also can trigger immune responses without any gastrointestinal symptoms. For example, British researchers reported in the journal *Neurology* that gluten sensitivity was the cause of headaches and the likely cause of inflamed brain tissue. Another study, published in the October 2001 *Rheumatology,* reported that 40 percent of subjects eating a gluten-free diet had a reduction in rheumatoid arthritis symptoms.

Specifically, celiac disease significantly increases the risk of a skin condition known as dermatitis herpetiformus, gastroesophageal reflux disorder, iron-deficiency anemia, irritable bowel syndrome, lactose intolerance, osteoporosis, and thyroid disease.

Leaky Gut Syndrome

Leaky gut refers to an abnormal permeability of the stomach and intestine wall, allowing incompletely digested proteins to enter the bloodstream. When such proteins move into the bloodstream, they trigger an immune response. Leaky gut is common in people with celiac disease, and it also may increase the likelihood of a variety of nongluten-related food allergies. A leaky gut can be caused by nutritional deficiencies, stress, stomach flu, antibiotics, and just about anything else that irritates the gut wall.

Nightshade Sensitivity

Some people, including an estimated 20 percent of people with rheumatoid arthritis, react to one or all nightshade foods, which include tomatoes, potatoes, eggplant, peppers, tomatillos, and tobacco (which is chewed or smoked rather than eaten). The reaction may be allergic in nature, or it may be that some people are very sensitive to small amounts of toxins in these foods.

How Common Are Food Allergies?

No one has precise numbers of the prevalence of food allergies and allergy-like sensitivities. Conventional allergists will often say they are rare, whereas physicians who routinely treat them may claim that 90 percent of people have at least one food allergy. The numbers of people with celiac disease are more precise, with the disease affecting about 1 in every 111 people—approximately 3 million Americans and 1 percent of the world population. Nonceliac gluten sensitivity, with often subtle symptoms, may affect half the population, according to some estimates.

The Inflammation Syndrome Connection

Food allergies with documented elevation of IgE and IgA antibodies reflect an immune system that has been unnecessarily stirred up. However, not all food allergies trigger these specific immune responses. It is possible that other types of immune reactions will eventually be identified, or that a person's symptoms occur through some other mechanism.

Allergic reactions may be greatest in one part of the body, such as in the gut or nasal area, but activated immune cells migrate throughout the body and frequently attack healthy cells, causing a wide variety of symptoms. In a sense, an allergic reaction shifts the normal biochemistry to a status resembling a military yellow or red alert. Such a heightened state boosts levels of other substances, such as adrenaline and the stress hormone cortisol. All of these stressful changes take a toll on the body and help deplete nutrients, so it is wise to reduce the symptoms of food allergies to relieve immediate discomfort and to lessen long-term wear and tear.

Standard Treatment

Conventional treatment of food allergens, when recognized, consists of avoidance.

Dietary Changes and Nutrients That Can Help

It is best to avoid foods that trigger allergic reactions. In addition, a rotation diet, in which the same food families are eaten only once every four days, may reduce the chances of future allergies developing. Avoiding an allergenic food for six months to a year sometimes allows the immune system to recover and not react to the problem food, as long as it is not consumed too often.

Several studies have found that low intake of fish and fish oils, or high intake of refined oils (such as margarine) are associated with a wide range of allergylike symptoms, rheumatoid arthritis, and asthma. Eating more fish and taking omega-3 fish oil supplements are likely to help, assuming that you are not allergic to the fish.

Sometimes concomitant allergies magnify a reaction. Concomitant allergies are a little like binary weapons, both parts being relatively innocuous until they are combined. Corn and banana, egg and apple, pork and black pepper, and milk and chocolate are common concomitant allergens. So are a variety of pollens and foods, such as ragweed and egg or milk, juniper and beef, elm and milk.

What Else Might Help?

Because damage to the gut wall is often involved in food allergies, several supplements might be useful in healing the digestive tract. Glutamine, an amino acid, plays important roles in gut-wall integrity. Probiotics, the term used to describe supplements of "good" gut bacteria, also might be helpful. Various digestive aid supplements, containing pancreatic or plant enzymes, might promote the complete digestion of food. Serenaid, a supplement that breaks down gluten, might help people deal with small and occasional amounts of gluten in the diet; it is available from Klaire Laboratories (800-859-8358).

When it is not possible to avoid a food, "neutralization" therapy might help. Minute amounts of an extract of an allergenic food are held under the tongue, from where they rapidly enter the bloodstream. It appears that the right dosage can inhibit the body's response to the allergen. The dosage has to be determined through *provocation* testing, which is done by a type of allergist known as a *clinical ecologist*.

Allergies, Inhalant

What Are Inhalant Allergies?

Inhalant allergies are immune system overreactions (hypersensitivities) to any type of otherwise innocuous substances, such as pollens, molds, and cat dander. These types of allergies typically elevate blood levels of immunoglobulin E (IgE), which is part of the immune response. Pollen allergies tend to be seasonal, causing reactions only when a specific grass or tree blooms, though some people react to many different pollens throughout much of the year. The most common symptom is rhinitis, which, in practical terms, means nasal inflammation, an itchy and runny nose, sneezing, and nasal congestion.

The term *atopic disease* is often used to describe inhalant allergies, but it is often inappropriate. Atopic suggests that such allergies are inherited. While people with allergies are likely to have allergic children, it is now common for children to develop pollen allergies although their parents and grandparents never experienced them.

Causes

When an immune system reacts to something, such as ragweed pollen, when it shouldn't, it is obvious that something serious has gone awry. Pollens or dander are misidentified by immune cells as threats, triggering a massive and physically uncomfortable response. While medical and drug researchers are trying to figure out the molecular details of what goes wrong, they miss the obvious: allergies, on the scale that they now exist, are a recent phenomenon. So what has changed?

Research conducted by Francis Pottenger, M.D., during the 1930s offers a clue about how modern dietary changes have led to significant increases in the prevalence of allergies. Pottenger conducted a variety of dietary studies on more than nine hundred cats. He found that when the quality of their diets declined, health problems developed and grew worse, with each subsequent generation eating the same poor diet. By the third generation 90 percent of cats eating poor diets had developed allergies and skin diseases (which were usually manifestations of allergy). Many vitamins and minerals are needed for normal functioning of the immune system, and suboptimal levels of nutrients and deficiencies impair the normal programming of immunity.

Pottenger found that this trend could be reversed in the second generation, but that it took four generations of normal feeding to once again yield healthy nonallergic cats. That reversal was not possible by the third generation of cats eating a nutritionally deficient diet. Furthermore, the cats became incapable of reproducing by the fourth generation, the last.

If you see parallels between the lives of Pottenger's cats and people today, you are on the right track. Based on the prevalence of allergies, many people (and families) are in the equivalent of second and third generations eating poor diets; one of every five American couples is infertile.

How Common Are Inhalant Allergies?

Inhalant allergies have become very common in Western industrialized nations and rare in less developed countries. Approximately 20 percent of Americans have allergies, which translates to almost 60 million people. As many as 17 million Americans also have nonallergic rhinitis, and 22 million have a combination of allergic and nonallergic rhinitis. Nonallergic rhinitis refers to the symptoms but without any identifiable allergic cause. According to Robert S. Ivker, D.O., of Denver, Colorado, 40 million Americans suffer from sinusitis, one manifestation of rhinitis.

The Inflammation Syndrome Connection

The first phase of allergic rhinitis involves sneezing and a runny nose after exposure to an allergen. This is followed by an increase in eosinophils, immune cells that promote inflammation, and, importantly, set the stage for a hair-trigger immune response after further exposures to the allergen.

Researchers believe that a shift in the ratio between two types of immune cells, Th_1 and Th_2 cells, which increases production of IgE and certain cytokines, predisposes people to allergies. But what causes the shift? The evidence is growing that a diet high in pro-inflammatory omega-6 fatty acids is largely to blame. Finnish researchers compared twenty allergic and twenty nonallergic mothers and found that both groups of women consumed the same amounts of omega-6 and anti-inflammatory omega-3 fatty acids in their diets. However, breast milk from the allergic mothers contained less of the omega-3 fatty acids, which would predispose their infants to allergies.

Long-term, inhalant allergies maintain a steady inflammatory state in the body, generating free radicals that further fuel inflammation. People with inhalant allergies often have food allergies as well. Allergies are a serious stress on the body, causing unnecessary wear and tear.

Standard Treatment

Avoidance of allergens is the best way not to have allergic reactions, but it is easier accomplished when the allergen is cat dander rather than pollen. Over-the-counter antihistamine products block allergy symptoms, but at a cost: drowsiness and an increased risk of cancer. Some prescription antihistamines (Claritin, Allegra, and Zyrtec) are safer than over-the-counter varieties. Immunotherapy—allergy shots—also can blunt symptoms, as can corticosteroid drugs.

Perhaps the best and safest over-the-counter allergy medication is cromolyn sodium, sold under the brand name NasalCrom. Cromolyn sodium is actually a synthetic flavonoid. It works by desensitizing cells in the nasal cavity that would otherwise react to an allergen and appears to have no systemic side effects, an effect that has similarities to the natural flavonoids in vegetables and fruit. NasalCrom is a nasal spray, and it is most effective when used several times a day, starting two weeks before pollen exposure. It also may help in dealing with allergies to cats and dogs. Other advantages to NasalCrom are that it is nonsedating and its activity appears limited to nasal tissues.

Nutrients That Can Help

Some physicians have become receptive to nutritional therapies because vitamin supplements relieved or eliminated their own allergies. For example, Robert Cathcart III, M.D., was impressed by how vitamin C supplements relieved his hay fever, and he went on to become one of the leading experts in the clinical use of vitamin C to fight infections.

A large variety of nutritional supplements might help, but you will have to experiment to find the best combination for your particular body and allergies. Vitamin C (1 to 5 grams daily), quercetin (300 to 1,000 mg daily), and omega-3 fish oils (1 to 3 grams daily) make a good start. Several B vitamins, including niacinamide, pantothenic acid, and vitamins B and B_{12}, also may help relieve allergies; a B-complex supplement may be better than individual supplements. Again, do whatever you can to reduce exposure, such as using air conditioning and high-efficiency air filters.

What Else Might Help?

Many people swear by honey as a way to reduce pollen allergies. It is very likely that honey produced in your region contains small amounts of pollen that serve as a "neutralizing dose," blocking larger amounts of pollen from triggering immune reactions.

Many foods seem to exacerbate allergic reactions to pollens, and it is probably worthwhile testing such foods by avoiding them for a week or so. Wheat, other grains, and dairy products, because of their own allergenic potential, often can aggravate pollen allergies.

Considerable research indicates that a disruption of the normal bacteria inhabiting the gastrointestinal tract can increase the likelihood of allergic sensitization during infancy. Taking antibiotic treatments for ear infections is a common method of destroying normal gut bacteria. Taking probiotic (good bacteria) supplements can reduce the damage when antibiotics must be taken.

Alzheimer's Disease

What Is Alzheimer's Disease?

Alzheimer's disease is the most common type of dementia. (The second most common form is caused by blood clots from ministrokes, a cardiovascular problem.) Alzheimer's is characterized by a serious impairment and worsening of memory, plus a decline in at least one other cognitive function, such as in perception or language skills. As Alzheimer's progresses, it leads to a loss of motor skills and reduced independence in daily activities, such as grooming and going to the bathroom.

Causes

Alzheimer's is characterized by deposits of beta-amyloid protein, as well as beta-amyloid tangles between brain cells. The beta-amyloid protein is believed, in some way, to choke brain cells.

How Common Is Alzheimer's Disease?

An estimated 4 million Americans have some degree of Alzheimer's disease. The Alzheimer Foundation projects that more than 14 million people will develop it by 2050, largely a consequence of 76 million aging baby boomers. Although these numbers may be inflated, the number of Alzheimer's cases is likely to increase because of the aging population and a decline in dietary quality.

The Inflammation Syndrome Connection

A major clue is that both animal and human studies have shown that use of ibuprofen, a common anti-inflammatory drug, reduces the risk of developing Alzheimer's disease. In animals the drug reduces the amount of beta-amyloid plaque. People who take ibuprofen are less likely to develop the disease.

Free radicals are known to stimulate the accumulation of beta-amyloid protein, and antioxidants have been suggested by Denham Harman, M.D., Ph.D., of the University of Nebraska, as one means of counteracting the process. Of course, free radicals promote the activity of adhesion molecules in inflammation. Unfortunately, it has been difficult for researchers to document the presence of specific immune cells in the brain, which would confirm the role of inflammation.

Standard Treatment

Several drugs are used to slow the progression of Alzheimer's disease, including selegiline. However, vitamin E appears to be slightly more effective than selegiline.

Nutrients That Can Help

The role of free radicals in promoting brain damage points to the potential benefits of antioxidant supplements. Indeed, a range of studies with cells, animals, and people have found antioxidants to be of benefit. The most dramatic study, published in the *New England Journal of Medicine,* found that very high doses of vitamin E (2,000 IU daily) extended the ability of late-stage Alzheimer's patients to care for themselves. Researchers are currently investigating whether the same dosage of vitamin E can slow or reverse the early stages of Alzheimer's. However, if your mind is in good shape, 400 to 800 IU is probably sufficient for long-term prevention.

A number of other antioxidant supplements might also be protective, including vitamin C, coenzyme Q_{10}, and alpha-lipoic acid. Specific dosages are hard to determine because of the limited amount of research on these antioxidants and Alzheimer's disease. Extracts of the herb Ginkgo biloba also might be beneficial, though the research has been conflicting. Ginkgo serves as both an antioxidant and as a dilator of blood vessels in the brain, improving blood circulation to neurons.

Some research indicates that the anti-inflammatory properties of omega-3 fish oils also can reduce the risk of neuroinflammation. Given the progressive nature of Alzheimer's disease, the emphasis should be on prevention or reversing its early stages. It is not likely that advanced Alzheimer's disease can be reversed because of extensive damage to brain cells.

What Else Might Help?

Several other nutrients also might protect against cognitive decline and Alzheimer's disease. Acetyl-L-carnitine, 2 grams daily, has been found to improve attention spans, long-term memory, and verbal abilities in some Alzheimer's patients. Phosphatidyl serine, a phosphorus-containing fat, is essential for the health of cell membranes, particularly brain cells. Dosages of 300 mg daily have been found helpful in improving memory, but 100 mg also might work in mild cases of memory impairment.

Difficulty concentrating—that is, fuzzy thinking—is often an early sign of diabetes. Elevated blood sugar levels and full-blown diabetes accelerate the aging process and, presumably, that of the brain as well. The Anti-Inflammation Syndrome Diet Plan is a low-glycemic, glucose-stabilizing diet, and it should improve glucose tolerance.

Arthritis, Osteoarthritis

What Is Osteoarthritis?

Of more than one hundred types of arthritis, osteoarthritis is by far the most common. Osteoarthritis refers specifically to a breakdown of the cartilage pad in at least one joint, such as the fingers, knees, or elbows. It also can affect the neck, hips, and lower back, even resulting in a decrease in height. These pads, known as articular cartilage, cushion the impact and lubricate the movement of bones in a joint. When articular cartilage is thin or completely gone, bones grind directly against each other. Signs of osteoarthritis include inflammation, swelling, pain, stiffness, and difficulty moving one or more joints. Nearly every person over age sixty has some degree of osteoarthritis, though the disease progresses at different rates from person to person.

Causes

For the most part, osteoarthritis is a disease of wear and tear; the more you use your joints, the more you lose them. Overuse, such as in athletics, and athletic injuries can accelerate the breakdown of articular cartilage. Sometimes immune cells inflaming tendons can spread out and affect a nearby joint.

Being overweight, even by as few as ten pounds, also can increase the risk of osteoarthritis. One reason is that the extra weight puts more stress on joints. Another is that fat cells secrete large amounts of pro-inflammatory interleukin-6 and C-reactive protein, which increase inflammation throughout the body.

An often overlooked cause is that relatively few people nowadays consume cartilage, which contains the building blocks of our own joints. In the past it was common to make soups using chicken or beef bones, with cartilage (and other nutrients, such as calcium) dissolving in the broth. Cartilage attached to the bones releases glucosamine and chondroitin, two important building blocks of our own cartilage. It is very possible that people would have less need for glucosamine and chondroitin supplements if they had regularly consumed homemade soups.

The omega-3 fatty acids found in fish oils inhibit some of the enzymes involved in breaking down articular cartilage, so eating less fish also may increase the risk of developing osteoarthritis. Allergylike food sensitivities also may influence symptoms of osteoarthritis. Exposure to allergens often varies, and this could explain why many arthritics feel better or worse from day to day.

How Common Is Osteoarthritis?

About three times as many women as men have osteoarthritis, and about one in every fourteen people (21 million in the United States) suffer mild to crippling symptoms. That number is expected to rise to 30 million by 2020. Overall, one in seven people has some form of arthritis, 40 million in the United States. That number is expected to increase to one in six by 2020.

The Inflammation Syndrome Connection

Immune cells are drawn to sites of injury, where they release powerful inflammatory compounds. Immune cells help clean up damaged cells, such as in torn ligaments, strained tendons, and flakes of bone and cartilage. Many mild injuries may not even be noticed, or their complete healing may be wrongly assumed. Injured tissue is more susceptible to repeated injury, and this situation may lead to chronic inflammation.

Standard Treatment

More than 250 different drugs are used to treat arthritis, including aspirin and other nonsteroidal anti-inflammatory drugs (NSAIDs), cortico-steroids, and Cox-2 inhibitors. All have undesirable side effects. Some NSAIDs, such as ibuprofen, actually increase the breakdown of cartilage. Replacements of hip and knee joints are surgical treatments for severe cases of osteoarthritis.

Nutrients That Can Help

For osteoarthritis, supplements of glucosamine and chondroitin, about 1,200 to 1,500 mg of each daily, have been shown to reduce pain and inflammation. One excellent study found that glucosamine supplements can help rebuild articular cartilage, and chondroitin appears to have some anti-inflammatory properties. (For more details, review chapter 10.) Vitamin C is needed for the formation of collagen and cartilage, as are manganese and sulfur. A minimum of 500 mg of vitamin C may be needed. Additional sulfur, also essential for cartilage formation, can be obtained in glucosamine sulfate, chondroitin sulfate, or methylsulfonylmethane (MSM), and small amounts of manganese can be obtained in a multimineral supplement.

What Else Might Help?

A variety of other nutrients, herbs, and habits also may reduce inflammation and pain associated with osteoarthritis. The least expensive change is to drink more water. According to Hugh D. Riordan, M.D., of the Center for the Improvement of Human Functioning International, Wichita,

Kansas, poor hydration is a common problem. Sufficient water intake helps cushion cells and tissues.

Vitamin D may indirectly reduce the risk of osteoporosis, according to research by Timothy E. McAlindon, D.M., a medical doctor and rheumatologist at Boston University Medical Center. Vitamin D is necessary for normal bone development, and low levels may affect bone structure and stability underneath the cartilage pads in joints.

Another study, by Margaret A. Flynn, Ph.D., professor emeritus at the University of Missouri, Columbia, found that supplemental vitamin B_{12} and folic acid could improve hand-grip strength in men and women with osteoarthritis of the hands.

The herb ginger also may be helpful. A study in *Arthritis & Rheumatism* found that patients taking a ginger extract benefited from moderate improvements in knee pain. The study confirmed ginger's use as an anti-inflammatory agent in Chinese medicine, dating back more than twenty-five hundred years.

Two topical treatments also can help. Several studies have found that creams containing capsaicin, the pungent component of hot peppers, can reduce the pain of osteoarthritis. Capsaicin blocks the transmission of pain chemicals to the brain. The effect appears to be strictly symptomatic, but other than a local sensation of heat, it is far safer than acetaminophen and other nonsteroidal anti-inflammatory drugs. Creams containing the herb arnica also may relieve joint pain.

Lastly, mild movement therapies such as walking, yoga, and swimming may improve flexibility and reduce pain. It is very important, however, not to overdo such exercises because they may further break down articular cartilage.

Arthritis, Rheumatoid

What Is Rheumatoid Arthritis?

Rheumatoid arthritis is an autoimmune disease, which means that the immune system mounts a full-scale attack on the body's own tissues. In rheumatoid arthritis the attack is centered on connective tissue near joints. Early symptoms include inflammation, pain, stiffness, tenderness, and swelling. However, this disease also has wide-ranging systemic effects including fever, reduced appetite, weight loss, and fatigue.

Rheumatoid arthritis is generally progressive—it gets worse with time. There may be periods of remission when symptoms decrease or even temporarily disappear. Long-term, it can be disfiguring and turn fingers into stiff, twisted digits. About 20 percent of people with rheumatoid arthritis develop lumpy nodules under the skin. In some cases it becomes completely disabling.

Causes

It is possible that some cases of rheumatoid arthritis are triggered by an immune response to a viral infection. Whatever the triggering event, the severity of the disease reflects a highly disturbed immune system that cannot distinguish friendly cells from foes. To many observers it looks as though immune cells are chasing after biochemical ghosts.

Considerable research has shown that people with rheumatoid arthritis are commonly deficient in multiple nutrients. These deficiencies can impair immune function, and the benefits of nutritional supplementation have been confirmed by numerous studies. Several cases of scurvy (extreme vitamin C deficiency) have been reported with rheumatism as the most obvious symptom. Low levels of vitamin C lead to a weakening of blood vessel walls, allowing red blood cells to leak into surrounding tissue, where they trigger an immune response. Vitamin C supplementation resolved the symptoms in these patients.

How Common Is Rheumatoid Arthritis?

An estimated 2.5 million Americans (about 1 percent of the U.S. population) have rheumatoid arthritis. It affects twice as many women as men.

The Inflammation Syndrome Connection

Levels of several pro-inflammatory cytokines—interleukin-1, interleukin-6, and tumor necrosis factor alpha—are typically elevated in people with rheumatoid arthritis. These cytokines instruct immune cells to unleash a powerful attack. The tenderness, pain, and swelling are by-products of chronic, intense inflammation.

Standard Treatment

Most medications—more than 250 different kinds—are designed to relieve pain. But none of them treat the underlying disease process.

Nutrients That Can Help

Many people benefit from the anti-inflammatory effect of omega-3 fish oils. However, it may take several months to see an improvement. A Scottish study of sixty-four men and women found that supplements containing about 3 grams of omega-3 fish oils daily resulted in a significant reduction of arthritic symptoms and less need to take conventional medications. Other research has shown that omega-3 fish oils reduce levels of the pro-inflammatory cytokines interleukin-1 and tumor necrosis factor alpha.

Gamma-linolenic acid (GLA), an anti-inflammatory omega-6 fatty acid, may be even more effective in rheumatoid arthritis. GLA boosts levels of anti-inflammatory prostaglandin E_1, which suppresses pro-inflammatory prostaglandin E_2. Human trials with GLA (approximately 1.4 grams daily) have shown consistent benefits over several months, reducing symptoms by roughly one-third to one-half. Of course, results will vary from person to person, and a combination of supplements will likely have greater benefits.

Increased intake of olive oil also can reduce symptoms of rheumatoid arthritis. Olive oil reduces the activity of adhesion molecules, which enable white blood cells to attach to and attack normal cells.

People with rheumatoid arthritis tend to have low antioxidant levels, and two studies so far have found that natural vitamin E supplements significantly reduce symptoms of the disease. The dosage used in these studies was relatively high, 1,800 IU daily. Vitamin E also lowers levels of interleukin-6 and C-reactive protein, both of which promote inflammation. Selenium, another antioxidant, also might help, but the research has not been consistent. The mineral boosts production of glutathione peroxidase, one of the body's main antioxidants.

People with arthritis have low levels of numerous other nutrients, such as vitamins B_2 and B_{12}, folic acid, calcium, and zinc. Deficiencies of folic acid and vitamin B_{12} are often exacerbated by methotrexate, one of the drugs used to treat rheumatoid arthritis. Methotrexate interferes with the metabolism of these two B vitamins.

What Else Might Help?

Many studies point to the apparent role of allergylike food sensitivities in rheumatoid arthritis. These adverse reactions to food can ramp up immune activity and inflammation. Dairy products and gluten-containing grains (such as wheat, rye, and barley) are among the most common food allergens, and studies have found that their avoidance eases arthritic symptoms, including morning stiffness and the number of swollen joints in many people, as well as reducing C-reactive protein levels. The elimination of allergenic foods may explain why fasting and gluten-free vegetarian diets help some people with rheumatoid arthritis.

According to Loren Cordain, Ph.D., a researcher at Colorado State University, lectins also might trigger symptoms of rheumatoid arthritis in some people. Lectins are a family of plant proteins found primarily in legumes, but also in wheat and rice. Like gluten, lectins may cause an inflammation of the gut, leading to a more generalized immune response. Temporarily avoiding lectin-containing foods may confirm a sensitivity to them.

Two additional supplements also might be of benefit: An animal study found that the antioxidant extract of green tea blocked the activity of several pro-inflammatory compounds, protecting against rheumatoid arthritis. Other research suggests that supplemental cetyl-myristoleate also might lessen symptoms of rheumatoid arthritis.

Asthma

What Is Asthma?

During asthmatic episodes, or attacks, the body's airways (bronchi and bronchioles, which deliver air to the lungs) overreact to pollen, cat dander, cigarette smoke, cold air, or other stimuli. The airway wall muscles begin to spasm, narrowing the opening and allowing less air to reach the lungs. An inflammatory response results in a rapid thickening of mucus, which further narrows the airway. An asthma attack may begin with wheezing, coughing, or shortness of breath; suffocation can occur in rare cases.

Causes

Ask ten different allergists about the cause of asthma and you may get twenty different explanations. A nearly mind-boggling number of causes have been proposed: dust, dust mites, cockroaches, house mice, wall-to-wall carpeting, central heating, gas stoves, overly sealed (insulated) buildings, candida yeast infections, pollen, and food allergies. In addition, some people blame urban air pollution. While air pollution certainly can trigger asthmatic attacks, urban air pollution has generally declined, while the number of people with asthma has increased. The same pattern is true with secondhand cigarette smoke, which can increase the risk of asthma in children—but fewer people are smoking, and the rate of asthma continues to rise. Others point the finger at the widespread use of antibacterial cleansers or antibiotics, both of which might reduce routine exposures to bacteria and interfere with the normal programming of immune systems.

All of the above factors can trigger asthmatic reactions in sensitive people. So can a host of other factors, including exercise, cold air, aspirin, sulfites (a preservative used in wines, beers, and some salad bars), and tartrazine (a yellow coloring used in some foods and drugs). In addition, emotional stress can induce asthmatic reactions in some people, and being overweight predisposes some people to asthma.

Like a fish that does not realize it is living in polluted waters, many people with asthma and many allergists don't understand that they are essentially swimming in a polluted diet. The modern diet, which is high in pro-inflammatory omega-6 and trans fatty acids and low in antioxidants, sets the stage for asthmatic reactions. In effect, asthma is one of many diseases of modern civilization and modern eating habits.

People with asthma tend to have higher than normal levels of free radicals, which stimulate inflammatory reactions and also indicate low intakes of antioxidant nutrients. Several studies have found that both children and adults have better lung function and are less likely to wheeze when they eat a lot of fruits and vegetables, the main dietary sources of antioxidants. Breast-feeding also may reduce the risk of asthma and other respiratory illnesses. J. Stewart Forsyth, M.D., of Ninewells Hospital, Dundee, Scotland, noted in the *British Medical Journal* that "nutritional deficiencies at critical periods of fetal and infant growth may induce permanent changes in physiological function."

Other research points to inadequate levels of anti-inflammatory omega-3 fish oils in the diet. A study of almost six hundred children by Ann J. Woolcock, M.D., of the Royal Prince Alfred Hospital, Australia, found that those who regularly ate fresh fish rich in omega-3 fatty acids had one-fourth the risk of asthma, compared with children who ate little or no fish. In a separate article, Jennifer K. Peat, Ph.D., a colleague of Woolcock's, noted that the increase of childhood asthma corresponded with a fivefold increase in the use of vegetable oils (rich in pro-inflammatory omega-6 fatty acids) and a shift to using margarine instead of butter. Similar changes have occured in New Zealand, England, and the United States.

How Common Is Asthma?

Asthma is the most common *obstructive airway disease*. Several decades ago, it was a rare respiratory disorder. Today it affects 17 million Americans, one-third of them children. Its prevalence in the United States has doubled since the 1970s, and African Americans and Hispanics experience particularly high rates of the disease. In Britain the incidence of asthma in children doubled during the 1990s.

The Inflammation Syndrome Connection

Asthma usually begins when the immune system becomes sensitized to an allergen, which may be a food, tobacco, proteins from cockroaches, or dander from pets. The immune system responds whether the trigger is a real threat or not, releasing a variety of inflammatory molecules. An upper respiratory tract reaction may cause little more than a runny nose (rhinitis), but asthma develops when the bronchi or bronchioles (which branch out from the bronchi) start overreacting to inflammatory molecules. One relationship is clear: the increase in asthma is related to the overall increase in allergies—that is, inflammatory reactions to generally innocuous substances.

Standard Treatment

A wide variety of medications are used to lessen asthmatic reactions, including corticosteroids and bronchial dilators. Most have long-term consequences. For example, corticosteroids increase the risk of cataracts and weak bones.

Nutrients That Can Help

Several studies have shown that large amounts of antioxidant nutrients can greatly reduce the frequency and severity of asthmatic reactions. Herman A. Cohen, M.D., of Rabin Medical Center, Israel, gave 2 grams of vitamin C or a placebo to twenty men and women, ages seven to twenty-eight, all with exercise-induced asthma. An hour after taking the vitamin or placebo, their lung function was measured as they walked or ran on a treadmill. Half of the patients had milder asthmatic reactions after taking the vitamin C, while those taking placebos experienced a significant decline in lung function.

Similarly, researchers at the University of Washington, Seattle, gave vitamin E (400 IU) and vitamin C (500 mg) daily to patients with asthma who were exposed to ozone (an air pollutant) and asked to run on a treadmill. After taking the antioxidants, the patients tolerated the ozone and exercise with considerably less breathing difficulty and, sometimes, with improvements in lung function.

Two studies have found that the antioxidants beta-carotene and lycopene, found in vegetables and fruit, can ease asthmatic reactions. Ami Ben-Amotz, Ph.D., of Israel's National Institute of Oceanography, and his colleagues measured lung function in thirty-eight people with asthma, then asked them to run on a treadmill. The subjects had an average decrease of at least 15 percent in their lung function. Next, Ben-Amotz gave them 64 mg of natural beta-carotene (derived from *Dunaliella* algae) daily for seven days. After taking the supplements (equivalent to about 100,000 IU daily), they went back on the treadmill. This time, twenty (53 percent) of the subjects had significant improvements in their postexercise breathing. In particular, these twenty patients initially had an average 25 percent decrease in lung function after exercising, but only a 5 percent reduction after taking beta-carotene supplements.

In the other study, Ben-Amotz asked twenty people with exercise-induced asthma to take either 30 mg of lycopene (the amount found in seven tomatoes) or placebos daily for one week. All of the subjects taking placebos had a 15 percent decline in lung function after exercising. But 55 percent of those taking lycopene had improvements in lung function after exercising.

Ozone, a common component of urban air pollution, is toxic to the respiratory system, and it increases the inflammatory response in people with asthma. However, in a study at the University of Washington, Seattle, supplements of vitamin E (400 IU) and vitamin C (500 mg) daily greatly improved breathing in seventeen adults with asthma after they were exposed to ozone.

In addition, research has found that omega-3 fatty acids—3 grams daily—can significantly reduce bronchial reactivity in asthmatic patients. Other studies have found similar benefits, though the results have not always been uniform. Rather than relying only on omega-3 fatty acids, people with asthma might have greater success by also taking gamma-linolenic acid, vitamin E, and other nutritional supplements.

What Else Might Help?

Many other nutrients help ease asthmatic reactions, and it is worth trying them—in addition to strictly following the Anti-Inflammation Syndrome Diet Plan. People with asthma commonly have low levels of magnesium, a mineral involved in more than three hundred biochemical processes in the body. Magnesium also is a mild muscle relaxant, so it may directly reduce the frequency and severity of reactions. Zinc and selenium also might be of benefit, along with quercetin (which inhibits some types of inflammation-promoting adhesion molecules) and the herb boswellia. A study published in the *Journal of Medicinal Food* reported that the herbal antioxidant Pycnogenol (1 mg per pound of body weight, up to 200 mg daily) improved lung function in patients with asthma. It is also important to maintain a normal weight, because overweight increases the risk of asthma. (See "Overweight and Obesity" in this chapter.)

Athletic and Other Injuries

What Are Athletic Injuries?

Athletic injuries can damage tissues so severely that they ultimately lead to chronic inflammation and pain and a complete breakdown of those tissues. The same can happen for any type of nonathletic physical injury as well, such as a broken bone from a fall or a muscle strain from lifting too heavy an object. Pain and discomfort long after an injury are signs of its incomplete healing.

Most athletic injuries and other types of physical injuries affect the skin, cartilage, muscles, and bones. Muscles strains and sprains, tendinitis, and bone fractures are the most common injuries. Repeated stress to the cartilage pads in joints, particularly in the knees, can weaken these cushions and set the stage for osteoarthritis. Physical stresses also may bruise internal organs such as the kidneys or the brain. For example, many boxers develop neurological damage years after they were fighting in the ring and absorbing punches. Even marathon runners exhibit elevated levels of inflammation-causing substances after a long-distance run.

Causes

Serious single injuries, repeated bruising, and overuse injuries are physical stresses to the body. They crush, tear, or break tissues, and healed tissue may not be quite as sturdy or resilient as tissue that has never been injured. Granted, accidental injuries are sometimes unavoidable, regardless of whether a person is a well-conditioned athlete or an average person who happens to trip over a crack in the sidewalk.

Injuries generate large numbers of free radicals released by activated white blood cells. Studies have found that broken bones and damaged cartilage increase free-radical levels, even without the presence of white blood cells. In addition, ischemic-reperfusion injuries also boost free-radical levels and tissue damage. Ischemia refers to a reduction of blood flow, often the first phase of an injury, which is followed by an influx of red blood cells; both phases generate large quantities of free radicals.

In general, the risk of injuries and painfully slow healing increases with age. Everyone knows that children tend to bounce back from injuries, but adults heal much more slowly. As was discussed earlier, our bodies experience an age-related deterioration. Bones, skin, and other tissues become thinner, and muscle mass declines—these are, after all, some of the signs of aging. It is important to keep in mind that fifty-year-olds don't have the physical attributes of twenty-five-year-olds. The chances of being injured can increase when a person denies the reality of aging and its concomitant decreases in strength, flexibility, reflexes, and coordination. When injuries occur, it is imperative that chronic inflammation be prevented and healing be supported nutritionally.

How Common Are Athletic Injuries?

Every person involved in athletic activities risks some type of injury. Professional athletes are conditioned and trained to minimize the risk of such injuries, but injuries still occur. For example, professional baseball pitchers usually rest for at least three days after starting a game. Weekend warriors, people who engage in sports only occasionally, are often neither conditioned nor trained. They run a high risk of developing overuse injuries, such as tennis elbow, golf elbow, or sore knees, as well as far more serious injuries. "Boomeritis," a term used to describe athletic injuries in the middle-age baby boomer generation, has increased dramatically in recent years. During the 1990s, medical office visits for boomeritis jumped by 33 percent among people between ages thirty-five and fifty-four. During the same time, emergency room treatment of sports-related injuries shot from 276,000 to 365,000 in the United States.

The Inflammation Syndrome Connection

Inflammation is the body's immediate response to injury. It enables a variety of blood cells to flood the site of the injury—platelets to stop bleeding, red blood cells to nourish healthy cells, and white blood cells to clear up damaged cells and fight infections. However, without adequate levels of many nutrients, healing cannot be completed and the inflammatory response cannot be turned off.

Standard Treatment

NSAIDs are commonly used to reduce inflammation and pain, but they can lead to excessive bleeding and ulcers. Some injuries must be treated surgically.

Nutrients That Can Help

Søren Mavrogenis, a physiotherapist in Copenhagen and the physical therapist for the Danish Olympic team, uses a combination of fatty acids and antioxidants to treat injuries among Olympians and other elite athletes. The fatty acids include omega-3 fish oils (706 mg daily), gamma-linolenic acid (670 mg daily), and modest amounts of antioxidant vitamins and minerals.

In one of several controlled studies, Søren and Norwegian physicians treated forty recreational athletes, men and women eighteen to sixty years old, with the fatty acid/antioxidant supplement or placebos for one month. All of the subjects had suffered overuse injuries in sports activities, experiencing chronic inflammation for at least three months before entering the study. In addition to the supplements and placebos, the subjects also received physical therapy. Nearly all of the participants had significant reductions in their inflammation and pain.

Exercise is well documented for increasing levels of free radicals, which can damage DNA. This DNA damage may account for the weathered looks of many serious athletes. Clinical trials have found that vitamin E supplements can reduce or prevent such DNA damage. Vitamin C quenches free radicals as well, and also is crucial for forming new collagen and cartilage during the healing process.

What Else Might Help?

Pycnogenol, a complex of natural antioxidants obtained from the bark of French maritime pine trees, has impressive anti-inflammatory properties. It also increases the body's synthesis of collagen and elastin, another tissue protein. Anthony Martin, D.C., of Montréal, has advised many professional Canadian athletes who have been injured. In one case, a hockey player who had injured his knee was told by his team's physician that he would probably need surgery and be on the sidelines for eight weeks. Martin recommended that the player take 400 mg daily of Pycnogenol. His knee stopped swelling, and after a week he no longer needed crutches.

He was also able to avoid surgery and was playing hockey again after just three weeks.

Several other nutrients may be especially helpful in healing injuries. Methylsulfonylmethane (MSM), 1,000 to 2,000 mg daily, has been found very effective in reducing muscle and joint pain. S-adenosyl-L-methionine (SAMe) stimulates the body's production of collagen. Both nutrients likely work at least in part because they donate sulfur to key biochemical processes. In addition, the B vitamins have an analgesic effect and are required for the production of new, healthy cells.

Cancer

What Is Cancer?

Cancer refers to the growth of abnormal cells, which can displace the normal cells composing tissues. Cancers are often distinguished by their ability to metastasize, spreading to and attacking other organs. There are many different types of cancer, but all arouse fear because of how they cut life expectancy and because of the pain associated with cancer and with conventional therapies (surgery, radiation, and chemotherapy). Although some cancers affect children, they are usually age-related: the older you are, the greater your risk of cancer. In general, cancers take years to develop, and many cancers go undiagnosed until autopsy.

Causes

Cancers are caused by mutations, or changes, in the deoxyribonucleic acid (DNA) that programs cell behavior. These mutations generally occur in two ways: through random transcriptional errors when cells normally replicate, and through free-radical damage to DNA. These errors permanently alter the cells' genetic instructions—analogous to being told to turn right on a street instead of left. The immune system recognizes and destroys most abnormal cells, but some are able to evade normal immunity. As a person gets older, a larger number of cell mutations and poor immune surveillance increase the likelihood of cancer.

How Common Is Cancer?

Cancer is the second leading cause of death in the United States and one of the most common causes of death worldwide. A little more than five hundred thousand Americans die of cancer each year. By far, cancers of the lungs and bronchi are the leading causes of cancer-related death in the United States, and they also are a common cause of death among non-smokers. Breast cancer in women, prostate cancer in men, and colorectal cancer are the next most common types of cancer.

The Inflammation Syndrome Connection

According to Bruce N. Ames, Ph.D., a leading cell biologist at the University of California, Berkeley, about 30 percent of all cancers are related to chronic inflammation or chronic infections. Both inflammation and infections generate free radicals, which can damage DNA, and the level of damage increases when these conditions are chronic. In addition, viruses also can mutate cells.

Standard Treatment

Conventional medical treatments of cancer are generally aggressive and designed to eradicate cancerous cells. They include surgical removal of the tumor mass or affected organ, radiation, and chemotherapy. Despite the many claims of advances in cancer treatment, the cure often seems worse than the disease. Indeed, an analysis published in the *Journal of the American Medical Association* found that improvements in the so-called five-year survival rate in cancer patients had more to do with better (earlier) diagnosis than with successful cures.

Nutrients That Can Help

Good nutrition and high intake of most micronutrients help preserve the integrity of DNA. Because of this, nearly every nutrient can play an important role in reducing the risk of cancer. However, some nutrients may be more important than others.

Antioxidant nutrients curb the activity of free radicals and, as a consequence, can reduce DNA damage. Selenium, part of the potent antioxidant glutathione peroxidase, has been shown to inhibit dangerous mutations to the flu and coxsackie viruses; vitamin E also prevents mutations to the coxsackie virus. Based on this research, it is highly plausible that selenium and vitamin E also might block virus-induced mutations that could give rise to cancer cells.

In general, vitamins E and C and flavonoids are potent antioxidants that can reduce DNA damage from various types of free radicals. Contrary to some news reports, vitamin C does not increase DNA damage or the risk of cancer. In one case, scientists corrected their warning and apologetically stated that vitamin C actually reduced DNA damage. Another study, performed in test tubes, showed no cancer-causing effect, though newsletter headlines claimed that vitamin C did.

Large dosages of vitamin C (10 grams or more daily) do have some benefit in treating cancer, particularly if the vitamin C is delivered intravenously. Many studies also have found that high-potency supplementation can extend the life expectancy of cancer patients, though these studies are often ignored by oncologists. In terms of prevention, vitamin E and selenium supplements are probably the best supplements for reducing the overall risk of cancer.

The B vitamins play crucial roles in the body's synthesis and repair of damaged DNA. Folic acid, vitamin B_{12}, vitamin B_3, and vitamin B_1 may be particularly important, especially in ensuring accurate gene transcription and repair. Some research also suggests that the omega-3 fatty acids reduce inflammation in the digestive tract and may reduce the risk of colon cancer.

Many anti-inflammatory nutrients have been directly linked to lower rates of specific cancers. For example, fish oils are associated with a lower risk of colon cancer. Lycopene lowers the risk of prostate cancer, and one study found that it reduced the size of prostate tumors in men scheduled for surgery.

What Else Might Help?

Cigarette smoke and other pollutants do their damage in large part by disrupting normal DNA transcription and by causing free-radical damage to DNA. Some of the free radicals may be part of the chemical pollutant, other free radicals may be produced when the liver tries to break down the pollutants. Thus, it helps to avoid tobacco smoke, live in a city that does not have serious air pollution, and to minimize exposure to cancer-causing chemicals at work and at home. If avoidance is not possible, the evidence suggests that supplemental vitamin E, selenium, and B vitamins—along with a diet with a diverse selection of vegetables—might rank toward the top of a cancer-prevention strategy.

Several aspects of diet are especially relevant in this context. First, high-fat diets promote the growth of many cancers, such as those of the breast and prostate. For prevention and during cancer treatment, it is worthwhile to reduce and, especially, to alter the ratios of specific types of fats. Several compelling studies have shown that fish oils have a cancer suppressive effect. In contrast, corn, safflower, and other vegetable oils high in omega-6 fatty acid promote the growth of cancers.

In addition, researchers at the University of Utah, Salt Lake City, had determined that diets high in trans fats are associated with significant increases in the risk of colon cancer. Given the fundamental roles of fatty acids in health, it would be prudent to avoid a synthetic fat that interferes with other fatty acids. Thus the ideal approach during cancer treatment might be to drastically reduce overall fat intake while emphasizing dietary fish and fish oil supplements. Under these circumstances it might also be best to avoid red meats and even to limit consumption of chicken and turkey.

Chronic Obstructive Pulmonary Disease

What Is Chronic Obstructive Pulmonary Disease?

Chronic obstructive pulmonary disease (COPD) is a chronic blockage of the airways, resulting from chronic bronchitis or emphysema. Chronic bronchitis is defined as a persistent cough with sputum, without a medically identifiable cause. Emphysema describes an enlargement of minute air sacs, called alveoli, and the destruction of their walls, which impair lung function. When the lungs cannot take in adequate oxygen, the body's cells become oxygen-deprived.

Causes

The leading cause of COPD is smoking, though extreme air pollution can degrade lung capacity. COPD may start to develop within five to ten years after a person starts smoking. Smoker's cough is one sign of COPD, as is the tendency for a head cold to move to the chest. By the time a person reaches his or her late fifties or early sixties, reduced lung function may result in shortness of breath, making washing, cooking, and dressing difficult.

How Common Is Chronic Obstructive Pulmonary Desease?

In the United States an estimated 14 million people have COPD, and approximately 104,000 die from it each year.

The Inflammation Syndrome Connection

Almost five thousand chemicals have been identified in cigarette smoke. Many of these release free radicals, which damage the proteins (elastin and collagen) that form the matrix of lung cells. In addition, white blood cells collect in aveoli, causing inflammation and further destruction of lung tissue. One cannot overstate the damaging effects of cigarette smoke—it is like living in a burning building and breathing in all of the noxious chemicals.

Standard Treatments

Prognosis and treatments are poor, though moderate exercise may improve overall quality of life.

Nutrients That Can Help

Compelling evidence indicates that a number of antioxidants and omega-3 fish oils may reduce the impact of air pollutants on lungs and help maintain normal lung function. This does not prove that these nutrients might help reduce the risk or severity of COPD. However, it is likely that these nutrients would exert some benefits in COPD, as long as they were consumed long before lung damage became irreversible.

N-acetylcysteine (NAC) is sometimes used by physicians to break up mucus in the lungs. Used on a long-term basis, NAC may help protect lung cells. A number of other antioxidants also might be helpful. Studies of smokers and beta-carotene have shown contradictory effects, but a modest intake of this carotene (10,000 IU or 6 mg) *in combination with other antioxidants,* such as vitamins E and C, is likely to be helpful. There appears to be a threshold of benefits from beta-carotene *in smokers,* so the above dosage should not be exceeded.

In a study of street workers in Mexico City, regarded as the most polluted large city in the world, men were asked to take 75 mg of vitamin E, 650 mg of vitamin C, and 15 mg of beta-carotene or placebos daily for 2½ months. When ozone levels were elevated, lung function in all of the men declined. However, men taking the antioxidant cocktail maintained better lung function throughout the study.

Still other research has found that lung function throughout life is related to intake of fruits and vegetables and high blood levels of antioxidants. One study found that vitamin E and beta-cryptoxanthin (found in papaya, peaches, tangerines, and oranges) were most strongly associated with good lung function.

James E. Gadek, M.D., of Ohio State University Medical Center, found that respiratory distress syndrome in hospitalized patients had significant improvements after they were fed a low-carbohydrate formula with vitamins E and C, beta-carotene, omega-3 fatty acids, and gamma-linolenic acid.

What Else Might Help?

There is no pill, natural or pharmaceutical, that will protect a person from the health effects of smoking. If you smoke, try your best to stop. Short of that, eat as many fruits and vegetables as you can. Smokers typically eat few fruits and vegetables, a rich and diverse source of antioxidant nutrients.

Coronary Artery (Heart) Disease

What Is Coronary Artery (Heart) Disease?

Coronary artery disease is characterized by a narrowing of the major arteries in the heart, a situation that leads to reduced blood flow and, in effect, slow starvation of cells forming the heart. The narrowing is caused by several factors, including lesions made up of cholesterol, abnormal growth of smooth muscle cells, and accumulated platelet cells. A heart attack occurs when a lesion grows large enough to completely block blood flow to the heart, or when part of a lesion breaks off and blocks an artery.

Causes

Theories describing the cause of coronary artery (heart) disease often become fashionable and then, after a number of years, unfashionable. Elevated levels of cholesterol were long seen as a major cause of heart and other cardiovascular diseases. The cholesterol theory oversimplifies the multifactorial causes of heart disease, and is being replaced by other theories, though you could not tell that by the large numbers of cholesterol-lowering drugs prescribed.

The two best explanations involve nutritional deficiencies and inflammatory injury to artery walls, and it is likely that both processes occur simultaneously. (They are not mutually exclusive.) One theory, proposed by Kilmer McCully, M.D., in 1969, argues that lack of certain B vitamins (chiefly folic acid and vitamin B_6) disrupts a fundamental biochemical process known as methylation. As a consequence, blood levels of homocysteine increase, damaging blood vessel walls. The body's response, meant to heal the damage, actually leads to the deposition of cholesterol and other substances.

The other theory, which dates back in part to clinical work by Evan Shute, M.D., in the 1940s and research by Denham Harman, M.D., in the 1950s, argues that oxidized LDL cholesterol is swallowed by white blood cells, which become lodged in the matrix of cells in artery walls. More recent clinical research by a variety of researchers, including Ishwarlal "Kenny" Jialal, M.D., of the University of Texas Southwestern Medical Center, Dallas, has clearly shown that *oxidized* but not normal LDL cholesterol is attacked and engulfed by white blood cells. What makes this research so intriguing is this: LDL is the medium through which fat-soluble nutrients such as vitamin E are carried in the blood. Oxidized LDL cholesterol is a sign of inadequate vitamin E intake (or, conversely, excessive intake of oxidized fats, such as in fried foods). Just as the B vitamins reduce homocysteine levels, so vitamin E reduces oxidation of LDL cholesterol.

How Common Is Coronary Artery (Heart) Disease?

An estimated 60 million Americans have coronary artery disease, and approximately 725,000 die each year from it, making it the leading cause of death in the United States. It is also the leading cause of death in Canada and England. Stroke accounts for another 116,000 annual deaths in the United States, with ischemic stroke (in effect, a "heart attack" in the brain) being the most common type.

The Inflammation Syndrome Connection

Research on the inflammatory nature of homocysteine and oxidized LDL cholesterol has helped establish coronary artery disease as an inflammatory process. The role of inflammation in heart disease has become better understood by the commercialization of a highly sensitive C-reactive protein (CRP) test and a shift in the medical perception of CRP. In the past high blood levels of CRP were seen as a marker of the body's inflammatory response after traumatic injury. The view today, which is more accurate, is that CRP is also a promoter of inflammation. It is a direct by-product of interleukin-6, perhaps the most inflammatory of the cytokines.

Although CRP levels reflect a general level of inflammation in the body, elevated CRP levels are a far more reliable predictor of heart disease than either cholesterol or homocysteine. People with high CRP levels are 4½ times more likely to experience a heart attack than are people who have normal levels. Arterial lesions containing CRP are unstable and highly likely to lead to breakaway fragments and clots. It is this relationship between CRP and heart disease, perhaps more than any other recent event, that has raised the medical consciousness of the role of inflammation in heart disease and other diseases.

Standard Treatment

The most common treatment for coronary artery disease consists of a class of cholesterol-lowering drugs known as statins. These drugs currently include Lipitor (atorvastatin), Mevacor (lovastatin), Pravachol (pravastatin), and Zocor (simvastatin). However, elevated cholesterol is more a symptom than a cause of coronary artery disease, so these and other drugs merely alter symptoms without addressing the underlying causes. Surgical treatments such as bypass and balloon angioplasty also are used to correct blocked arteries but do not change the underlying disease process.

Nutrients That Can Help

Many nutrients inhibit the inflammatory process in blood vessel walls and provide a variety of improvements in heart function. Several B vitamins lower homocysteine levels and appear to reduce the risk of heart attack. One study, published in the November 29, 2001, *New England Journal of Medicine,* found that modest supplements of folic acid, vitamin B_6, and vitamin B_{12} significantly lowered homocysteine levels and clearly reversed coronary artery disease in heart patients. Reducing homocysteine levels eliminates a major cause of blood vessel inflammation.

As discussed in chapter 9, vitamin E supplements lower CRP levels and, several clinical trials have found, reduce the risk of heart disease and heart attack. Vitamin E also reduces the tendency of LDL cholesterol to oxidize, which in turn keeps white blood cells from attacking LDL. In addition, vitamin E prevents the stiffening of blood vessel walls (endothelial dysfunction), which reduces blood flow and increases the risk of heart disease. Vitamin E also turns off the gene that programs the growth of excess smooth muscle cells, which also narrows blood vessels.

The omega-3 fatty acids found in fish oils and other sources, have diverse benefits to the health, stemming in part from their anti-inflammatory and cytokine-modulating properties. Research has found that the omega-3 fatty acids can reduce heart irregularities known as cardiac arrhythmias and also can lower blood pressure. In 2001 Danish researchers reported in the *American Journal of Cardiology* that heart patients with extensive narrowing of blood vessels had elevated levels of CRP and had low levels of omega-3 fatty acids. Supplements of omega-3 fatty acids should always be taken with vitamin E to protect them against oxidation.

Vitamin C and the B vitamin niacin (a form of B_3, which causes a temporary flushing sensation) have been found to lower cholesterol levels and to lower levels of lipoprotein (a), a cholesterol fraction that increases the risk of heart disease. In addition, magnesium plays a crucial role in heart rhythm, and supplements can sometimes reduce arrhythmias.

What Else Might Help?

It is of utmost importance to follow a diet that emphasizes nutrient density, such as the Anti-Inflammation Syndrome Diet Plan, which emphasizes fish, lean meats, and large amounts of fresh vegetables. Diets high in refined carbohydrates, sugars, and partially hydrogenated vegetable oils set the stage for insulin resistance and overweight, which increase the risk of pre- and full-blown diabetes and heart disease. Such a dietary approach, combined with anti-inflammatory nutritional supplements, also should reduce the severity of phlebitis, varicose veins, and blood pressure.

Finding some means of stress reduction or stress management is important as well. Stress raises levels of cortisol, which in turn boosts insulin levels—contributing to an increased risk of both abdominal obesity and heart disease. Removing yourself from the stress, even temporarily, can have an extraordinary effect. Consider a daily walk (which also lowers glucose and insulin levels), meditation, a hobby, recreational reading, or sightseeing as stress-reducing activities.

Dental Inflammation

What Is Dental Inflammation?

Three common dental disorders involve significant levels of inflammation: gingivitis, periodontitis, and temporomandibular joint (TMJ) syndrome. Chronic gingivitis refers to inflammation in the gum tissues visible near teeth. If your gums bleed when you floss or brush your teeth, there is a good chance that you have gingivitis. Periodontitis describes inflammation that is much deeper and involves the supporting bone of the teeth, and it is often missed in casual examinations. Periodontitis erodes the bone forming teeth. TMJ syndrome is generally recognized as a misalignment of the temporomandibular joint, located near the ears, which hinges the jawbone to the skull. This misalignment generates free radicals, which can fuel inflammation.

Causes

Each of these disorders has a different cause. Gingivitis results in large part from poor dental hygiene, which allows plaque-causing bacteria to proliferate and attack the gums. Periodontitis is associated with a different type of bacteria, but it is also often an age-related condition because some bone loss increases with age. TMJ syndrome is generally considered a consequence of malocclusion (crooked teeth). However, educator and author Malcolm Riley, D.D.S., of Tucson, Arizona, believes that TMJ syndrome is caused largely by stress, which leads to TMJ muscular spasms and pain.

How Common Is Dental Inflammation?

Dental caries (cavities) and periodontitis affect nearly every person at some point in life. For example, three out of four people develop some degree of gum disease by age thirty-five. The American Dental Association estimates that 10 million people in the United States might suffer from some degree of TMJ disease.

The Inflammation Syndrome Connection

In gingivitis, inflammation develops in response to bacterial infiltration of the gums. Similarly, in periodontitis, the breakdown of bone triggers an inflammatory response, which leads to additional destruction of bone. The inflammatory response activates a number of pro-inflammatory cytokines, which tell more white blood cells to get involved. If these cytokines leak into the bloodstream—a very likely event—they can prompt white blood cells throughout the body to react. In TMJ syndrome the sheering of bone generates large numbers of free radicals, which amplify pain and promote inflammation. All of these disorders are made significantly worse by smoking, which directly exposes oral tissues to large quantities of free radicals and which depletes antioxidants such as vitamin C.

People with periodontitis have a higher than normal risk of heart attack and stroke; people with any of these conditions commonly have elevated levels of C-reactive protein, a sign of inflammation. In addition, people with diabetes and rheumatoid arthritis—diseases with strong inflammatory components—have a higher risk of developing periodontitis and gingivitis.

Standard Treatment

Conventional dentistry takes a mechanical approach to what is a biological issue. Many dental procedures entail digging into tissues, filing away teeth, and building new structures. For example, the standard treatment for periodontitis in the United States is to clean teeth and then to cut away inflamed tissue. This contrasts with the approach of European dentists, who clean teeth and then allow the tissues to heal over many months. For gingivitis, conventional treatments involve better oral hygiene. TMJ disease is often corrected with a plastic cover over the teeth to separate the upper jaw and the lower jaw.

Dentists know that nonsteroidal anti-inflammatory drugs (NSAIDs) such as ibuprofen can slow the loss of bone in periodontitis. So this question arises: Why not use natural anti-inflammatory nutrients? Unfortunately, the answer is that most dentists are probably less knowledgeable than most physicians about the importance of nutrition in health.

Nutrients That Can Help

For long-term improvements in dental health, it is essential that you start with diet. Nearly everyone is taught that sugar-laden foods feed the bacteria that cause cavities. It is not as well known that sugary foods increase gingival inflammation. Cutting consumption of sugary foods and soft drinks reduces gingivitis, just as increased intake of protein and lower consumption of refined carbohydrates, combined with a multivitamin/multimineral supplement, reduce gingivitis.

Vitamin C intake also is important. In one study researchers found that intake of 65 mg of vitamin C daily eased gingival inflammation and bleeding, compared to when subjects received only 5 mg daily. However, much larger dosages (605 mg daily) led to even greater improvements in gingivitis and bleeding.

Low vitamin C intake is related to larger periodontal "pockets" (spaces around teeth where bone has been lost). While there are strong parallels between symptoms of gingivitis and periodontitis and the dental ramifications of scurvy (an extreme life-threatening deficiency of vitamin C), there also are major differences. In scurvy, bleeding from the gums is common, and vitamin C can reduce it. However, scurvy does not lead to the formation of fibrous scar tissue deep inside the gums, a sign of periodontitis. In addition, lower levels of inflammation are found in periodontitis than in scurvy.

Two other nutrients play key roles in controlling dental inflammation. In an animal study, vitamin E supplements reduced bone loss, very likely because it reduced inflammation. In several small human trials topical application of coenzyme Q_{10}, a vitaminlike nutrient, greatly improved periodontitis. To achieve the same benefits, break a soft gelatin capsule of CoQ_{10} (30 to 100 mg), massage its contents into the gums, and swallow the remainder.

What Else Might Help?

Although there has not been any research on the protective roles of omega-3 fish oils or gamma-linolenic acid in dental inflammation, supplements would likely have benefits. In addition, zinc supplements might promote healing of injured tissues. Calcium and magnesium might help maintain normal bone, and one study has found that glucosamine and chrondoitin reduce symptoms of TMJ disease when the joint is affected.

None of this information should negate the value of oral hygiene, but the best hygiene cannot make up for a poor diet and insufficient anti-inflammatory nutrients. Daily flossing and brushing along with periodic professional cleanings should be part of the best approach to dental health.

Diabetes

What Is Diabetes?

Diabetes is characterized by chronic elevated levels of blood sugar (glucose) and insulin. Glucose is the body's principal fuel, and insulin helps shuttle it into cells where it is burned for energy. However, high glucose levels are toxic to the kidneys, and diabetes is associated with a significantly increased risk of heart disease, cancer, kidney failure, blindness, and other diseases. In essence, diabetes accelerates the aging process, so diseases associated with old age occur during middle age.

Causes

Although glucose is blamed for many of the complications of diabetes, growing evidence also points to insulin. For example, people with diabetes who receive large amounts of insulin injections develop vascular disease more rapidly and extensively than do people who use less insulin.

Compelling research suggests that insulin is the oldest, or one of the oldest, hormones in living creatures on Earth. As such, its role is far more fundamental than simply regulating blood sugar levels. It turns on and off various genes and increases the production of body fat and, under different conditions, muscle.

What messes up things? People evolved eating low-carbohydrate foods, which only moderately raise glucose and insulin levels. The consumption of refined carbohydrates and sugars rapidly boosts glucose levels, and the body responds by secreting large amounts of insulin to move the glucose from the blood to cells. However, after a number of years of dealing with large amounts of glucose, cells become resistant to insulin's actions, with the consequence being chronic elevation of both glucose and insulin levels. Insulin resistance is the chief characteristic of diabetes.

Some genetically related groups of people, such as Native Americans, are especially sensitive genetically to insulin resistance and diabetes. But this genetic propensity only means that they develop the disease sooner rather than later when exposed to modern Western-style food. Genes aside, the real cause of type 2 (adult-onset) diabetes is dietary.

How Common Is Diabetes?

Full-blown adult-onset diabetes affects an estimated 15 million Americans, about half of whom have not been officially diagnosed with the disease. (Juvenile-onset diabetes is an autoimmune disease that is rarely reversible.) However, as many as 70 million Americans have some degree of insulin resistance or Syndrome X. Syndrome X refers to a cluster of insulin resistance, high blood pressure, abdominal obesity, and elevated cholesterol and triglycerides. (For more information see my previous book *Syndrome X.*) Basically, anyone eating the typical American diet is consuming foods that increase the risk of insulin resistance, Syndrome X, and diabetes.

The Inflammation Syndrome Connection

High levels of glucose autooxidize—that is, start a chain reaction that produces large amounts of free radicals and "advanced glycation products," both of which damage the body. Free radicals stimulate inflammatory responses and, in this way, people with diabetes develop high levels of inflammation. This situation has been well documented in several studies that have found sharp elevations of CRP and interleukin-6 in people with diabetes. Because of the ability of inflammatory cytokines to stimulate one another, people with diabetes typically have a strong undercurrent of inflammation, which increases the risk of other diseases, such as heart disease.

Standard Treatment

Glucose-lowering drugs such as metformin are usually prescribed to people with adult-onset diabetes. In severe cases insulin injections might be added to help lower glucose levels. As you might expect, side effects are common. Metformin interferes with the body's use of B vitamins, and insulin increases body fat, blood pressure, cholesterol levels, and arterial disease.

Nutrients That Can Help

Many supplements can lessen the inflammation in diabetes, but in this case, supplements can be like bailing water in a sinking boat: It is essential that the underlying diet be corrected.

That said, a key objective of supplementation should be to lower glucose levels and improve insulin function, which should in turn reduce inflammation. The chief supplements for improving glucose tolerance and insulin function are alpha-lipoic acid, chromium picolinate, vitamin E, vitamin C, and silymarin (an antioxidant extract of the herb milk thistle). If you are taking any drug for controlling glucose, be aware that your medication requirements may decrease.

Alpha-lipoic acid, a natural substance made by the body and found in beef and spinach, is used extensively in Germany to treat diabetic nerve disorders. In daily dosages of 600 mg it can improve insulin function and lower glucose levels in people with diabetes. It also is a powerful antioxidant.

A lack of chromium results in diabetes-like symptoms. Not surprisingly, therefore, supplements of chromium picolinate, a common form of chromium, have been shown to improve insulin function and lower glucose levels. Sometimes the effects can be significant after several months. In one U.S./Chinese study diabetic subjects were described as having a "spectacular" improvement after taking 1,000 mcg daily of chromium picolinate for several months. Diachrome, a proprietary combination of chromium picolinate and biotin, a B vitamin, have been shown to further enhance glucose control.

Vitamins E and C improve glucose tolerance and have the added benefit of lowering levels of CRP and interleukin-6. The effect of these vitamins on easing diabetic complications may be greater than their glucose-lowering properties.

Silymarin can have significant glucose-lowering effects in people with diabetes. An Italian study found major improvements in blood sugar levels and many other symptoms of diabetes after patients took silymarin supplements for one year.

By their nature, antioxidants have anti-inflammatory properties. Some antioxidants also influence the production of cytokines, so they reduce inflammation via another means. Based on insulin's fundamental role in biology, it is likely that the hormone controls the activity of some pro-inflammatory cytokines. It is worthwhile targeting a fasting glucose of between 75 and 85 mg/dl and a fasting insulin under 7 mcIU/ml.

What Else Might Help?

A person with diabetes must recognize that he or she has a potentially terminal disease, but one that usually can be modified and even reversed through diet. A relatively low glycemic diet, such as the Anti-Inflammation Syndrome Diet Plan, can moderate the spikes in glucose and insulin that result from refined carbohydrates and sugars. Protein will stabilize glucose and insulin levels, and the fiber in vegetables will have a similar effect because it blunts the absorption of carbohydrates.

It would be worthwhile as well for people with adult-onset diabetes to undergo testing for allergylike food sensitivities. For example, in one case, a person had no significant rise in glucose after eating ice cream, but had a several hundred point increase in glucose after having Scotch whiskey. A rise or decline of more than 50 points (mg/dl) in one hour is a sign of serious glucose-tolerance problems.

Gastritis, Ulcers, and Stomach Cancer

What Are Gastritis, Ulcers, and Stomach Cancer?

Gastritis refers to an inflammation of the stomach wall, as well as of the uppermost part of the small intestine, the duodenum. An ulcer, such as a peptic ulcer, is a lesion on the wall of the stomach. The most serious ulcers form deep craters or bleed. Gastric cancer is a growth of abnormal cells on the stomach wall. Sometimes, but not always, gastritis will evolve into an ulcer and both conditions increase the risk of gastric cancer.

Causes

For many years physicians believed that gastritis was the result of excess stomach acid, and drug treatments were designed to reduce the secretion of gastric juices or to make them more alkaline. In 1983 researchers identified a type of bacterium, *Helicobacter pylori,* in the stomach, and in the 1990s it was recognized as the leading cause of gastritis, ulcers, and stomach cancer. Conventional treatment now focuses on antibiotics and drugs that reduce the secretion of gastric juices.

However, there is a wrinkle to this story. With the successful use of antibiotics in eradicating *H. pylori* infections, a new leading cause of gastritis and ulcers has emerged: nonsteroidal anti-inflammatory drugs (NSAIDs) such as aspirin, ibuprofen, and coxibs. All NSAIDs, including the so-called Cox-2 selective drugs, disrupt the activity of cyclo-oxygenase-1 (Cox-1), an enzyme critical for fatty acid production and for maintaining the health of the stomach wall.

How Common Are Gastritis, Ulcers, and Stomach Cancer?

Gastritis affects roughly 3 million Americans, and an estimated 5 million people have gastric ulcers. Although stomach cancer does not garner many headlines, it is the second most common fatal cancer in the world, and in most countries the five-year survival rates are less than 20 percent. Chronic *H. pylori* infections boost the risk of stomach cancer by up to 80 percent.

The Inflammation Syndrome Connection

H. pylori irritates the stomach wall, but the immune response to this infection may wreak most of the damage. White blood cells are mobilized to the site of the infection, where they release free radicals and pro-inflammatory eicosanoids such as prostaglandin E_2. *H. pylori* is often highly resistant to this immune response, which can inflame the stomach wall and may eventually lead to an ulcer. Free radicals damage the DNA in stomach wall cells, increasing the chance of mutations, some of which could seed cancers.

The high levels of free radicals in the stomach rapidly deplete antioxidant levels in gastric juices and the wall, and numerous studies have found that gastritis and gastric ulcers are associated with low levels of vitamins E and C and beta-carotene. The situation is made worse when people consume relatively few fruits and vegetables, the principal dietary sources of antioxidants. In a Scottish study, researchers reported that *H. pylori* infection interfered with the body's utilization of vitamin C. When people infected with *H. pylori* ate few fruits and vegetables, their vitamin C levels dropped to one-third less than normal. Another study, conducted at the University of Auckland, New Zealand, found that people with *H. pylori* infections had only one-fifteenth the vitamin C in their gastric acid, compared with healthy subjects. Similar research has found that *H. pylori* compromises levels of vitamin E and the carotenoids, a situation that increases the risk of nearly every disease.

Standard Treatment

Antacids and drugs that alter the osmotic flow are commonly prescribed for gastritis and ulcers. A course of antibiotics is typically prescribed for people with gastritis or ulcers caused by *H. pylori* bacteria. Gastric cancer is treated with surgery or radiation.

Nutrients That Can Help

An impressive body of research, including clinical trials, has found that antioxidants strongly influence whether an *H. pylori* infection leads to gastritis, ulcers, or stomach cancer. Antioxidants can sometimes eliminate an *H. pylori* infection, though it is probably more judicious to use them in conjunction with antibiotics.

The most dramatic study investigated both antioxidant supplements and antibiotic therapy. Pelayo Correa, M.D., of Louisiana State University, New Orleans, asked 631 people with precancerous changes in their stomach-wall cells to take 30 mg of beta-carotene (50,000 IU) or 2 grams of vitamin C daily, a combination of both antioxidants, or a placebo for six years. Some of the subjects also underwent standard two-week antibiotic treatment for *H. pylori,* and others received both antioxidants and antibiotics. Changes to the gut were examined through endoscopy or biopsy after three and six years.

Correa found that three treatments—beta-carotene, vitamin C, and antibiotics—resulted in significant reversals of the precancerous stomach cells. In the treatment of nonmetaplastic atrophy, one type of precancerous condition, people receiving beta-carotene, vitamin C, or antibiotics were about five times more likely to improve than those receiving no treatment. Similarly, people with intestinal metaplasia, another type of precancerous condition, were almost 3½ times more likely to improve. In both cases the benefits of beta-carotene edged out vitamin C, and vitamin C edged out antibiotics. A combination of beta-carotene and vitamin C provided no additional benefits. However, 15 percent of the people taking antioxidants alone (no antibiotics) were cured of their *H. pylori* infection.

Two other studies have found that vitamin C supplements are beneficial. In a small trial sponsored by the World Health Organization, researchers gave 5 g of vitamin C daily for four weeks to thirty-two people with chronic gastritis and *H. pylori* infections. The supplements eradicated *H. pylori* infections in 30 percent of the patients. In Italy fifty-eight patients were treated with antibiotics, followed by either 500 mg of vitamin C daily for six months or no further treatment at all. Precancerous gastric cells were reversed in about a third of the patients taking vitamin C. In contrast, only one patient (technically 3.4 percent) from the other group improved.

What Else Might Help?

Other antioxidants also may offer protection against *H. pylori* infections and their consequential damage to the stomach. Among these are the herb Ginkgo biloba and garlic. Lycopene, a carotenoid that gives tomatoes their red color, has been associated with a relatively low risk of stomach cancer, though this association does not directly prove prevention. In addition, animal experiments suggest that food allergies also might irritate the stomach and lead to gastritis and ulcers.

An estimated 30 percent of people over age sixty-five suffer from atrophic gastritis, a chronic inflammation of the stomach associated with a wasting away of stomach tissues. The condition sharply increases the likelihood of vitamin B_{12} deficiency, which is significant because low levels of these vitamins can cause senile symptoms. It is important to keep in mind that the risk of atrophic gastritis does not suddenly appear at a certain age, but that it is a consequence of more subtle changes to stomach tissue and function. Although research in this area has focused on vitamin B_{12}, it is likely that atrophic gastritis and other forms of gastritis interfere with the absorption of many other nutrients. In addition, antiulcer drugs that inhibit the secretion of gastric juices could conceivably increase the long-term risk of atrophic gastritis.

Hepatitis

What Is Hepatitis?

Hepatitis literally means liver inflammation. It is usually, though not always, caused by a viral infection. Symptoms of acute hepatitis, which generally lasts fewer than six months, tend to appear suddenly and include fever, nausea, vomiting, and a general feeling of being ill. Many cases of acute hepatitis evolve into chronic low-grade liver infections.

Sometimes people with chronic hepatitis may be asymptomatic, and at other times they may experience extreme fatigue and loss of appetite. In both acute and chronic hepatitis liver enzymes become elevated—one sign of liver disease. Noninfectious hepatitis may result from drug or alcohol abuse. Often, the stress of hepatitis reduces levels of glutathione, one of the body's principal antioxidants, which is made in the liver. The viral and inflammatory stresses, combined with low glutathione levels, compromise liver function and may lead to cirrhosis or liver failure.

Causes

Viral hepatitis is caused by one of several viruses that attack this organ. The different types of hepatitis are referred to by a letter, as in hepatitis A or hepatitis B. Transmission of the different viruses occurs in a variety of ways. For example, hepatitis A is usually transmitted through fecal contamination of food, whereas hepatitis B is typically transmitted through sexual contact or shared needles. Hepatitis C is passed through blood, such as through shared needles or through pre-1991 blood transfusions. There are still other forms of hepatitis. One laboratory indication of hepatitis infection is an elevation in liver enzyme levels.

How Common Is Hepatitis?

Hepatitis C has received the lion's share of attention in recent years, and an estimated 4 million Americans have chronic hepatitis C infections. Many people have the disease without symptoms, and it may take decades of chronic hepatitis for it to become clinically apparent. Approximately ten thousand Americans die each year as a result of hepatitis C infections.

The Inflammation Syndrome Connection

Inflammation is the body's normal response to infection. But in chronic infection, the sustained immune activity may cause as much damage as, if not more than, the infection itself. From a biological standpoint, inflammation is very costly—stressful—to an organ. The liver is the body's largest organ, and it functions as a chemical processing plant, building needed molecules and breaking down toxins. This is a complex and diverse job, and the stress of a liver-specific infection is tantamount to a worker strike. When tissue damage and scarring become extensive, cirrhosis or liver failure may be the end result. Hepatitis results in more cases of liver failure than any other cause.

Standard Treatment

The most common pharmaceutical treatment is interferon, a synthetic version of a natural immune compound. However, interferon is expensive and frequently results in flulike symptoms that last for months.

Nutrients That Can Help

Burton M. Berkson, M.D., Ph.D., of Las Cruces, New Mexico, has found that a combination of three liver-supporting nutrients can control and reduce symptoms of hepatitis C. These nutrients are alpha-lipoic acid (discussed in chapter 11); selenium (also discussed in chapter 11); and silymarin, an extract of the herb milk thistle.

In the 1970s and 1980s Berkson used large doses of alpha-lipoic acid to treat *Amanita* mushroom poisoning, which often precipitates liver failure and death. Alpha-lipoic acid boosts the liver's production of glutathione, which aids the breakdown of *Amanita* toxins and promotes the synthesis of new liver cells. Similarly, selenium is needed for the liver to make several glutathione peroxidase compounds, all potent antioxidants. The herb milk thistle has been used for thousands of years as a liver tonic, and its silymarin extract is now recognized as a powerful antioxidant.

As with *Amanita* toxins (and many other toxic substances), the liver carries the burden of breaking down the poisons. Berkson has found that the combination of alpha-lipoic acid (600 mg daily), selenium (400 mcg daily), and silymarin (900 mg daily) is especially effective in lowering liver enzymes and restoring liver function.

What Else Might Help?

If you received a blood transfusion before 1991, when blood banks began testing for hepatitis C, it might be worthwhile to be tested. Even if the test provides bad news, it enables you to take steps to deal with the infection instead of allowing it to quietly run its destructive course.

Infections

What Are Infections?

Infections result from an attack on the body by pathogenic (disease-causing) bacteria, viruses, parasites, or prions. There are many ways to group infections, but for our purposes it is best to view them as either acute or chronic. Acute infections occur suddenly, such as in the case of colds and flus, followed by recovery. Chronic infections such as hepatitis or HIV/AIDS last many years and may be the ultimate cause of death. That said, acute infections can be very dangerous in themselves—the flu kills approximately twenty thousand Americans each year.

Causes

Most pathogens need a warm body to flourish. When they enter the body, typically through the mouth or the nose, and sometimes via the blood (such as through a cut or a transfusion), they trigger an immune response designed to destroy bacteria or virus-infected cells. However, many viruses and parasites can evade the immune response. A person's ability to resist infection, as well as to moderate symptoms of the infection, relates in large part to the health and efficiency of the immune system. The state of one's nutrition has a direct bearing on immune efficiency.

How Common Are Infections?

Everyone contracts an infection from time to time, whether it's a cold or an infected cut. Worldwide, infections have always been and are still the leading cause of death. If all of the infection-caused deaths in the United States were combined, they would add up to the third leading cause of death there, after heart disease and cancer.

The Inflammation Syndrome Connection

The immune system's inflammatory response is designed to kill pathogens. In colds, flus, and other acute infections, inflammation accounts for many of the symptoms, such as rhinitis, tenderness, and aches and pains. The consequence of this inflammation may last beyond the actual infection. As one example, Robert Cathcart III, M.D., of Los Altos, California, has pointed out that the stress of a cold or flu can lead to symptoms of an extreme vitamin C deficiency. That lack of vitamin C limits the body's ability to "clean up" excess free radicals produced by the immune system. These unquenched free radicals can cause considerable wear and tear on the body.

In many respects chronic infections, whether low-grade (such as parasitic infections) or more serious infections (such as HIV/AIDS), are more insidious. They force the immune system to remain at a heightened state of stressful activity, draining many of the body's nutritional and biochemical reserves. For example, people with HIV/AIDS often experience chronic diarrhea, which is likely the result of inflammatory bowel disease. The diarrhea limits absorption of essential nutrients, and high levels of vitamins and mineral supplements may be needed to achieve normal blood values.

Standard Treatment

Most over-the-counter treatments relieve symptoms, but often with undesirable side effects. For example, antihistamines may reduce nasal congestion, but they cause drowsiness and, long-term, they may increase the risk of cancer. Antibiotics can kill many types of pathogenic bacteria, but they disrupt some aspects of immunity and cause gastric disturbances. Some antiviral drugs reduce flu symptoms, but so far not to the extent of vitamin C or N-acetylcysteine (NAC). More powerful antiviral drugs can cause genetic damage.

Nutrients That Can Help

In general, the supplements that reduce symptoms of colds and flus can, in higher dosages, reduce symptoms and extend the lifespan in people with much more serious infections, such as HIV/AIDS. These nutrients do not have direct antiviral activity. Rather, they enhance the immune system's ability to confront the infection, as well as to prevent nutritional deficiencies that further compromise health.

Beginning in the 1970s Robert Cathcart III, M.D., started using large amounts of vitamin C, orally and at times intravenously, to treat patients with a variety of infections, including colds, flus, mononucleosis, hepatitis, and HIV/AIDS. Sometimes the dosages are truly massive, such as 100 grams or more daily. Cathcart found that people usually can tolerate large oral amounts of vitamin C without developing diarrhea when they are ill. As people recover, such large dosages of vitamin C become excessive and cause diarrhea, a sign that the dosage should be reduced. However, huge dosages of vitamin C may not always be necessary. In a review of twenty-one studies on vitamin C and the common cold, Harri Hemila, Ph.D., a professor at the University of Helsinki, Finland, found that 2 to 6 grams of vitamin C daily reduced the duration and severity of symptoms by about a third.

NAC is a potent antioxidant that, despite an unpleasant sulfur odor, has a significant effect on the symptoms and course of infections. It may, in fact, be superior to vitamin C. In a study of 262 elderly people, supplements of 600 mg of NAC daily reduced the occurrence of flu symptoms by two-thirds, and many people with laboratory-confirmed flu infections had no symptoms at all. In addition, researchers at Stanford University have reported that high dosages of NAC significantly extend the life expectancy of AIDS patients.

NAC also can help people with sepsis and septic shock. Sepsis, an infection of the blood, often pushes hospitalized patients to a life-or-death situation—not by a pathogen but by an overwhelming immune response to the infection. Researchers reported in the journal *Chest* that NAC reduced recovery times in patients with septic shock. NAC works in part by boosting glutathione, the most powerful of the body's own antioxidants. Selenium, part of the antioxidant enzyme glutathione peroxidase, increases survival among patients with a condition that has similarities to sepsis, severe system inflammatory response syndrome.

What Else Might Help?

To reduce the risk of contracting colds and flus, it is important to exercise caution when interacting with infected people. For example, wash your hands after touching a person (or touching objects the person has recently touched) who has such an infection. To reduce your risk of HIV and some types of hepatitis, avoid unprotected sexual contact or other exchanges of body fluids, such as through the use of unsterilized syringes.

Supplements of the herb echinacea stimulate immunity and appear to boost resistance to infections. It is possible that, as with NAC, echinacea does not protect against infections so much as it enhances immunity and renders symptoms negligible. Similarly, one clinical study unexpectedly found that people taking vitamin E supplements had 30 percent fewer colds. Lozenges containing zinc, a mineral needed for immunity, can significantly reduce cold and flu symptoms in many people, though the clinical findings have been mixed. The list of nutrients can go on, but it is important to remember that any deficiency impairs many aspects of health, including the degree of symptoms during an infection.

In children food allergies can increase the risk of ear infections. Allergies lead to fluid retention in the ears (which do not drain as well in infants and children as they do in adults), forming a breeding ground for bacteria. Eliminating the most likely food allergens, such as dairy and wheat products, can reduce the risk of ear infections.

Reduce the inflammatory stress caused by both acute and chronic infections. By doing so, you reduce the long-term damage—wear and tear, if you wish—from activated immune cells acting against their host.

Inflammatory Bowel Syndrome

What Is Inflammatory Bowel Syndrome?

Ulcerative colitis and Crohn's disease are the two types of irritable bowel syndrome (IBS). Both ulcerative colitis and Crohn's disease have similarities, and often it is difficult to distinguish between the two. As a general rule, ulcerative colitis is an inflammation limited to the wall of the colon (bowel). Its symptoms include abdominal cramps, fever, and bloody diarrhea. Similar symptoms, generally affecting the ileum (a portion of the small intestine) and without blood in the stools, are generally suggestive of Crohn's disease.

Causes

Officially, medicine does not know the cause of ulcerative colitis and Crohn's disease. However, the fact that IBS affects the digestive tract strongly points to an interaction with food.

How Common Is Inflammatory Bowel Syndrome?

An estimated 500,000 to 1 million Americans have either ulcerative colitis or Crohn's disease. People of Jewish descent are more likely than Gentiles to develop IBS.

The Inflammation Syndrome Connection

The abdominal cramps, which may come on suddenly, are spasmodic responses to an irritant. Various pro-inflammatory cytokines are elevated in people with IBS. The combination can lead to a "leaky gut" in which undigested food proteins move into the blood, causing a broader immune response.

Standard Treatment

A variety of drugs, including corticosteroids, may be prescribed for IBS. The role of diet is often ignored.

Nutrients That Can Help

It should come as no surprise that anti-inflammatory omega-3 fatty acids are helpful in relieving IBS. In a study published in the *New England Journal of Medicine,* researchers described how they gave 500-mg fish oil capsules or placebos daily to thirty-nine patients with Crohn's disease for one year. Only 28 percent of the people taking fish oil capsules had relapses of Crohn's disease, whereas almost two-thirds of those taking placebos experienced relapses. A much higher dose—7 to 15 grams daily—might prove more helpful.

Low levels of antioxidants also might hinder the body's ability to ease the inflammation. Canadian researchers have reported that people with Crohn's disease have elevated levels of "oxidative stress," a sign of inadequate antioxidants—even when symptoms are controlled by medication. For example, compared with healthy subjects, people with Crohn's disease had low selenium levels.

What Else Might Help?

It is essential that a person with IBS investigate the possibility of food sensitivities. The most likely dietary culprits are gluten-containing foods (wheat, rye, barley, and nearly every type of processed food) and dairy products. Eliminating these foods should improve symptoms within one to two weeks, if they were a cause of IBS.

One recent report by French researchers found that half of a group of 171 patients with Crohn's disease had elevated levels of homocysteine, a sign of folic acid and vitamin B_{12} deficiency. This does not necessarily mean that these B-vitamin deficiencies cause Crohn's disease, though they could be involved. Rather, the deficiencies may be a consequence of Crohn's disease that, over many years, could increase the risk of heart disease or stroke.

Lupus Erythematosus

What Is Lupus Erythematosus?

Lupus erythematosus is an autoimmune disease, meaning that the inflammation-causing immune cells attack the body's own tissues. It can affect different parts of the body, such as the skin, joints, kidneys, lungs, and cardiovascular system, and cause a wide variety of symptoms. Some cases are very mild, whereas others may be disabling or fatal. Ninety percent of people with lupus experience inflammation of their connective tissue, with symptoms often similar to rheumatoid arthritis, another autoimmune disease. Other common symptoms include rashes, sensitivity to sunlight, and kidney disorders.

Causes

No one really understands the cause or causes of lupus. Fever is common at its onset, suggesting that a bacterial or viral infection initiates the immune response (although inadequate vitamin B_1 also may cause fever). The hormone estrogen may influence lupus because it is most often diagnosed in women between their late teens and thirties. However, a hormonal link is tempered by the fact that estrogen therapies have not been useful as a treatment. It is conceivable that a woman's immune systems is simply biologically different in some ways from that of a man.

How Common Is Lupus Erythematosus?

Lupus affects approximately 1.6 million people in the United States, ten times as many women as men.

The Inflammation Syndrome Connection

As with other inflammatory diseases, particularly rheumatoid arthritis and multiple sclerosis, some factor or event turns immune cells against their host. Periods of remission are common, though lupus symptoms and tissue damage typically become worse with time.

Standard Treatments

Conventional treatments are intended to reduce inflammation and include corticosteroids as well as a variety of other immune-suppressing medications.

Nutrients That Can Help

Omega-3 fatty acids and vitamin E may help in controlling lupus. The evidence is more derivative than direct, based on the anti-inflammatory nature of these nutrients. A clinical trial published in *Arthritis and Rheumatism* found that large dosages of the hormone dehydroepiandrosterone (DHEA) may be beneficial. Supplements, which are available at health food stores, reduced the frequency of flare-ups. However, DHEA should be used under a physician's guidance.

One intriguing European study, published in *Phytotherapy Research,* found that supplements of the flavonoid-containing Pycnogenol significantly reduced markers of inflammation and disease activity in patients with lupus. Patients taking corticosteroids to suppress inflammatory symptoms benefited from greater reductions in symptoms after adding 120 mg daily of Pycnogenol, and they also had reductions in their sedimentation rate, a general indicator of inflammation. It is possible that grape seed extract and other flavonoids might be beneficial as well.

What Else Might Help?

While there is no clinical evidence to document its usefulness, it might be worthwhile to adopt (at least for a few weeks), a Paleolithic-style diet similar to the Anti-Inflammation Syndrome Diet Plan, as well as eliminating nightshade plants (such as tomatoes, potatoes, peppers, and eggplants). Such a diet provides high-quality protein and antioxidant-rich vegetables and fruit. At the same time such a diet eliminates calorie-dense carbohydrates, highly refined cooking oils, and trans fatty acids.

In addition, it might be helpful to take vitamin D (400 to 800 IU daily) supplements. Researchers at the University of Utrecht, Netherlands, reported that vitamin D deficiency is common among patients with lupus, either because they spend little time in the sun or because of how some medications interfere with the vitamin.

Multiple Sclerosis

What Is Multiple Sclerosis?

Multiple sclerosis (MS) is generally considered an autoimmune disease, in which immune cells attack the myelin sheaths wrapped around nerve fibers. Sclerosis is the medical term for lesion, and in MS multiple scar-like lesions form on the myelin, which is akin to the plastic insulation surrounding electrical wires. When the myelin becomes inflamed, it literally begins to fray, short-circuiting nerve signals and leading to the disease's physical and neurological symptoms.

Different MS symptoms are related to the location of specific nerve damage. They can take the form of extreme fatigue, weakness, a lack of balance, difficulty walking, double vision, speech problems, and depression.

Causes

Officially there is no known cause of MS. However, it is clearly related to an immune response that goes seriously awry. This immune reaction might be triggered by allergylike sensitivities, viral attack, physical injury, or any number of other insults, but the sustained damage appears related to the immune system. Although people with MS may have periods of remission, symptoms typically become worse—and crippling—over the years. On average, the life expectancy of people with MS is about a fourth less than that of people without the disease.

How Common Is Multiple Sclerosis?

MS affects an estimated 350,000 to 500,000 Americans. For reasons that remain mysterious, it strikes more women than men, most often between ages twenty and forty, and people of northern European descent (in contrast to Asians and Africans). According to a study at the University of California, San Francisco, the stress of daily hassles and major life events can exacerbate MS symptoms.

MS researchers have long recognized that the incidence of MS generally increases farther north and south from the equator, correlating to less sunlight. Sunlight activates the body's production of vitamin D, and people living farther from the equator would, over the course of a year, make less vitamin D. This relationship doesn't confirm that a lack of vitamin D increases the risk of MS. But there are other tantalizing data. According to a report by C. E. Hayes, Ph.D., and his colleagues at the University of Wisconsin, Madison, vitamin D can prevent experimental autoimmune encephalomyelitis, the mouse version of human MS.

The Inflammation Syndrome Connection

In autoimmune diseases most tissue damage is caused by immune cells rather than the event (if it is even identifiable) that triggered the immune response. For example, a form of the herpes virus known as *human herpes virus 6* seems to promote MS flare-ups, though most people harbor the virus without developing the disease.

What causes the immune overreactivity? It often seems to be related to a lack of anti-inflammatory nutrients in the diet. The modern diet, with a lopsided intake of fats, particularly highly refined fats and oils, may set the stage for MS in genetically susceptible people.

Although the prevalence of MS increases at extreme northern and southern latitudes, people living along the coast of Norway and throughout Japan have a relatively low incidence of MS. Such populations eat large amounts of fish, which are rich in anti-inflammatory omega-3 fatty acids.

Standard Treatment

Medications include short-term use of corticosteroids to suppress immune activity as well as interferon.

Nutrients That Can Help

Physicians at Trondheim University Hospital, Norway, have reported that 0.9 gram daily of omega-3 fish oil supplements significantly reduced MS symptoms in sixteen patients. In general, gamma-linolenic acid, found in borage seed oil, evening primrose oil, and olive oil enhance the anti-inflammatory effects of omega-3 fatty acids, so a combination of supplements might be ideal.

The perplexing increase in MS in extreme northern and southern regions might be explained by inadequate vitamin D. The body makes vitamin D when exposed to sunlight, but extreme latitudes have long winters and relatively few daylight hours. Recent research by Colleen E. Hayes, Ph.D., a biochemist at the University of Wisconsin, Madison, has shown that vitamin D suppresses the autoimmune reaction underlying MS. In experiments with laboratory mice Hayes found that vitamin D raised levels of two anti-inflammatory compounds (interleukin-4 and transforming growth factor beta-1) and stopped the progression of the animals' version of MS.

Brief exposures to sunlight (fifteen to thirty minutes daily) stimulate the body's production of vitamin D, and people living or working in sunny climates may produce more than 10,000 IU daily. According to Hayes, a very high dose—4,000 IU daily—may be required to achieve normal levels of the vitamin among people who do not receive sunlight.

This dose is ten times higher than the Recommended Daily Value, and because large, chronic doses of vitamin D may be toxic, it's best to take it under the guidance of your physician. He or she can monitor your blood levels of vitamin D, which should be about 100 nmol/L (nanomoles per liter of blood).

What Else Might Help?

Several other nutrients might reduce MS symptoms. Antioxidants such as vitamin E, flavonoids, and alpha-lipoic acid might ease inflammation. Vitamin B_{12} also might be of value. Several years ago E. H. Reynolds, M.D., of King's College Hospital, London, found that MS patients were almost always deficient in vitamin B_{12}, which is needed for normal nerve function. Japanese researchers gave MS patients huge dosages of vitamin B_{12} (60 mg, not mcg, daily) for six months. Their visual and auditory symptoms improved, but muscle function did not.

Because dietary fats have been so skewed by refining and processing, it might be worthwhile to adopt a Paleolithic-style diet similar to the one described in this book. Emphasizing anti-inflammatory fats and studiously avoiding pro-inflammatory trans fatty acids might have benefits.

Overweight and Obesity

What Are Overweight and Obesity?

By clinical definition, a person is obese when he or she is thirty or more pounds over his or her ideal weight. Simply being overweight is characterized by being a few pounds to up to thirty pounds over his or her ideal weight. Of course, a well-trained muscular person might be incorrectly considered overweight because muscle tissue is more dense and heavy than fat tissue. Therefore, accurate assessments should calculate fat-to-muscle or hip-to-waist ratios. From a practical standpoint, a look in the mirror can make much of the testing unnecessary. Most people who are overweight or obese know that they are, though they might want to deny the obvious.

Causes

Overweight and obesity usually are diseases of overeating, although metabolic factors affect some people. The traditional view is that people gain weight when they consume more calories than they burn. This is partly true because many people are not as physically active as their ancestors, but it fails to explain everything.

Often ignored is that diet can serve to exacerbate or moderate a preexisting metabolic disorder. In addition, the source of calories is at least as important as the overall quantity of calories. That is because protein is far less likely than carbohydrate to be stored as fat. In general, high-sugar and high-carbohydrate foods trigger a stronger insulin response, compared with protein-rich foods, and insulin helps promote the accumulation of body fat. High-sugar and high-carbohydrate foods also tend to be short on fiber, protein, omega-3 fatty acids, and vitamins and minerals that either buffer the absorption of carbohydrates or aid in the body's metabolism of them.

Several animal studies have found that some dietary fats are more likely than others to become body fat. For example, some research shows that consumption of monounsaturated fat results in less body fat than does saturated fat, even when both provide the same number of calories. Similarly, evidence suggests that consumption of omega-3 fatty acids, calorie for calorie, might result in relatively less body fat.

How Common Are Overweight and Obesity?

The prevalence of obesity and overweight have, without exaggeration, skyrocketed in recent years. In 2001 David Satcher, M.D., then surgeon general of the United States, described it as an "epidemic." He predicted that the health consequences of overweight and obesity would soon overtake the effects of tobacco. Thirty-one percent, or almost one-third, of North Americans are now obese. They are part of the 65 percent—two-thirds—of North Americans who are now overweight. The number of overweight children also is disturbing. Estimates of overweight children range from 13 to 20 percent.

These increases in weight result largely from the increased consumption of junk foods consisting chiefly of refined sugars, carbohydrates, and fats. A major source of dietary sugar is soft drinks, which the consumer-oriented Center for Science in the Public Interest has described as "liquid candy." A 64-ounce bottle of any calorically sweetened (in contrast to artificially sweetened) soft drink contains approximately ½ cup of sugar! Children have essentially been weaned on soft drinks and calorie-dense fast-food restaurant fare. "Super-size" meals lead to super-size children and adults.

Some physicians have noted that the rapid increase in the prevalence of overweight followed public health recommendations in the 1980s to eat low-fat diets. Low-fat diets usually translate into high-calorie, high-carbohydrate diets that, again, scrimp on protein, vitamins, and minerals.

Being overweight is the number one risk factor for developing adult-onset diabetes, and overweight children and teenagers now account for half of all new diagnoses of diabetes. The prevalence of type 2 diabetes among children has increased by an estimated fifteen to twenty-five times since 1980. Being overweight also increases the risk of hypertension, heart disease, gallstones, colon cancer, and (in men) stroke.

The Inflammation Syndrome Connection

The high-sugar and high-carbohydrate diets that lead to obesity raise glucose levels, and elevated glucose spontaneously generates large numbers of free radicals. These free radicals stimulate the inflammatory response, which can increase the risk of coronary artery disease, cancer, Alzheimer's, and many other diseases. In addition, abdominal fat cells secrete large quantities of pro-inflammatory interleukin-6 and C-reactive protein. In overweight and obese people both of these substances help maintain a state of chronic inflammation.

Increases in body fat are often associated with disturbed hormone levels such as elevated cortisol and insulin and decreased thyroid hormones. Sometimes figuring out which came first is like the chicken-or-the-egg story. However, being overweight leads to hormonal shifts that make it easy to gain still more weight. Because of their cell-regulating actions, it is very likely that weight-promoting hormones increase the activity of pro-inflammatory cytokines.

Standard Treatment

Conventional wisdom holds that people should eat fewer calories and exercise more to lose weight. Exercise helps because it creates more muscle cells, which burn calories for energy. But compelling research indicates that calories from protein and good fats are far better than those from carbohydrate-rich foods such as pasta, bread, and pizza. It makes no sense to build a diet around empty calories. Instead, follow a nutrient-dense diet such as the plan described in this book.

Nutrients That Can Help

The many fat-burning, fat-blocking, or carbohydrate-blocking supplements sold may help a small number of people, but they skirt the bottom-line issue: people cannot take a simple pill to compensate for bad eating habits. At best it is naive to believe that supplements (or medications) can combat a diet full of high-calorie, high-carbohydrate refined foods.

Persuasive research by Harvard Medical School scientists has shown that diets rich in refined carbohydrates and carbohydrate-dense vegetables and grains increase CRP levels and inflammation. In the study, potatoes, breakfast cereals, white bread, muffins, and white rice were most strongly associated with elevated CRP levels. As with diabetes, it is essential that a person exercise the responsibility to choose healthier foods, such as those recommended in the Anti-Inflammation Syndrome Diet Plan. Such a diet should emphasize nutrient-dense lean meats (such as chicken and turkey), fish, and vegetables, while deemphasizing calorie-dense sugary foods and grain-based carbohydrates. The simple rule is to get as much diverse nutrition as possible in every bite of food. That is more easily accomplished with fish and vegetables than with pasta or pizza.

What Else Might Help?

A number of supplements might enhance weight reduction, but they are by themselves unlikely to burn off pounds of fat. Such supplements as alpha-lipoic acid, coenzyme Q_{10}, and carnitine play key roles in the cellular breakdown of glucose and fat. Supplements containing ephedra, a stimulant, may help as well—but they carry risks that include higher levels of anxiety and nervousness and increased blood pressure, and I do not recommend them.

Skin Disorders

What Are Skin Disorders?

Your skin is your body's largest and most direct interface to the world around you. As such, it is exposed to a wide variety of insults, including air pollution, chemicals, sunlight, bacteria, and viruses. Under these circumstances, a vast number of conditions can cause transitory or chronic inflammatory skin disorders. Only a few examples of inflammatory skin disorders will be described here as proof that anti-inflammatory nutrients can be beneficial. Among these disorders are contact dermatitis, sunburn, psoriasis, and eczema.

Causes

Dermatitis literally means skin inflammation, and the term is usually interchangeable with eczema. Both are generally descriptions, not specific diseases. Dermatitis can take a variety of forms anywhere on the body, including itchiness, inflammation, swelling, and flaking skin. Many people consider dandruff a hair-related disorder, but it is actually a skin condition known as seborrheic dermatitis.

Contact dermatitis is often caused by direct handling of an irritating chemical. The body can often adapt to the exposure, which is what happens to people regularly working with chemicals. However, many people pay a physiological price—complete intolerance of the chemical—after a number of years. Some types of contact dermatitis are also caused by specific naturally occurring compounds in a variety of foods. Dermatologists refer to this as "balsam-related contact dermatitis." The term comes from a plant extract called balsam of Peru, which contains allergenic substances, which are also found in tomatoes, citrus, cola drinks, chocolate, and various spices (including vanilla).

Mild sunburn, known as erythema, is actually an inflammation of the skin. It is caused by damage from ultraviolet (UV) rays in sunlight, which split apart water molecules in cells and create free radicals. Tiny blood vessels rupture, and white blood cells respond to the damage. Regular sunburn or more severe sunburn can increase the long-term risk of skin cancers. That is because free radicals damage the DNA in skin cells.

Psoriasis is a chronic skin disease that often begins during a person's teenage years. It is characterized by thick, red skin patches. These patches are covered by white or silvery scales. These skin lesions itch, burn, crack, and sometimes bleed. About 15 percent of people with psoriasis also have arthritic joints, a condition known as psoriatic arthritis. Psoriasis tends to be worse during the winter months, when the air is drier and people have less exposure to sunlight.

Finally, wrinkling reflects age-related changes in the skin, including free-radical damage to the proteins forming skin and a thinning of the skin. Wrinkling can be accelerated by smoking and by excessive exposure to the sun.

How Common Are Skin Disorders?

Everyone experiences some type of dermatitis from time to time. Psoriasis, one of the most common chronic skin disorders, affects more than 7 million Americans. Many people enjoy the darker complexion afforded by a tan, but sun worshipers usually develop premature wrinkling and an increased risk of skin cancer, consequences of skin-cell damage from ultraviolet light.

The Inflammation Syndrome Connection

Research by Lester Packer, Ph.D., and Jens Thiele, M.D., of the University of California, Berkeley, has shown that the skin contains a reservoir of fatty acids and antioxidants. When the skin is exposed to ozone (a common air pollutant) or UV radiation, free radicals are generated, depleting these antioxidants and oxidizing fatty acids. UV-generated free-radical damage to the skin occurs in only two minutes. The inflammatory response occurs much as it does elsewhere in the body, but it is far more visible. A blistering sunburn (or skin burns from chemicals and fire) is a sign of much more severe skin damage and cell death. Also important to note, skin levels of antioxidants decline with age, possibly increasing the rate of damage.

Standard Treatment

Treatments for psoriasis include corticosteroid drugs, both oral and topical. Corticosteroids also are used topically to treat many types of skin inflammation. Sunscreens can block some exposure to ultraviolet radiation, but they are often improperly used. For example, sunscreens protect the skin for short periods, and they are easily washed off.

Nutrients That Can Help

The classic signs of fatty acid deficiency (omega-6, omega-3, or both) are dry and flaking skin. Such symptoms can develop when people are malnourished or eat low- or zero-fat diets. Eating fish and taking fish oil capsules can provide omega-3 fatty acids, and olive oil is an excellent source of omega-9 fatty acids. Adequate amounts of omega-6 fatty acids can be obtained in olive oil and raw nuts such as almonds, or pumpkin seeds.

Several antioxidants have been shown to be helpful in reducing the effects of sunburn. Combined with omega-3 fatty acids, antioxidants can likely ease other forms of skin inflammation through an inside-out approach: take oral supplements and use a topical cream with antioxidants. Vitamin E is the body's principal fat-soluble antioxidant, meaning that it protects against free-radical damage in fatty parts of cells such as membranes. Topical applications are well absorbed through the skin, with some of the vitamin also entering general circulation. In addition, topically applied vitamin E blocks UV damage to DNA. In a recent study Bernadette Eberlein-König, M.D., of the Technical University of Munich, measured how daily oral supplements of vitamin E (1,000 IU) and vitamin C (2,000 mg) increased resistance to UV rays. She found that subjects taking the vitamins were about 34 percent more resistant to sunburn, compared to people taking placebos.

Vitamin C also can reduce the damaging effects of UV radiation. A study by Steven S. Traikovich, D.O., of Phoenix, Arizona, found that a vitamin C–containing lotion was able to reduce fine wrinkles, roughness, and skin tone compared to a similar lotion without the vitamin. Vitamin C is essential for the body's production of collagen and elastin, two of the key proteins forming skin. In addition, several studies have found that beta-carotene supplements enhance the protective effects of sunscreen, illustrating the benefits of an inside-out approach to skin care.

Pycnogenol, a complex of antioxidant flavonoids extracted from the bark of French maritime pine trees, has been shown to reduce inflammation and, specifically, protect skin cells. Laboratory experiments have shown that Pcynogenol decreases the activity of two genes, calgranulin A and B, which are overactive in psoriasis and some other skin disorders. Pycnogenol decreased the activity of calgranulin A and B by twenty-two times. Other researchers have shown that Pycnogenol helps prevent the breakdown of elastin from inflammation and free radicals.

What Else Might Help?

Like many herbs, chamomile *(Matricaria chamomilla)* is rich in antioxidants. In Germany it has a rich history of use in treating skin disorders and also is found in many modern cosmetics. Allergist Holger Biltz, M.D., of Bad Honnef, Germany, found that a chamomile-containing cream reduced reddening after UV exposure and reduced skin roughness. One high-quality line of chamomile-containing skin products is CamoCare, available at many natural foods stores and pharmacies. Green tea also is a powerful antioxidant and may be helpful in some skin disorders.

A wholesome diet, similar to the Anti-Inflammation Syndrome Diet Plan, can help preserve the skin. Australian researchers have reported that people eating diets with large amounts of olive oil, fish, and vegetables experienced less facial wrinkling compared with people who ate more red meat, processed deli meats, soft drinks, and pastries.

Lastly, it is paramount not to smoke tobacco products and not to be in the sun long enough to get sunburned. Smokers develop a particular type of facial wrinkling, which is related to their premature aging in general. Approximately fifteen minutes of sun exposure daily are sufficient for the body to make large amounts of vitamin D, but not enough to result in sunburn (for most individuals). Longer sun exposure should be accompanied by the use of sunscreen or UV-blocking clothing.

Staying Healthy
for Life

The prevalence of inflammatory diseases has clearly increased over the past several decades. Part of this increase is related to the overall aging of the population. After all, inflammation is one consequence of age-related wear and tear on the body. Millions of people already suffer from a variety of inflammatory diseases. And in the United States alone, almost 80 million baby boomers (born between 1946 and 1963) are entering middle age, a time when even the healthiest people are likely to notice some deterioration in their health.

However, I am convinced that the increase in inflammation has accelerated as a consequence of eating a poor or unbalanced diet, a situation others have described as malnutrition on a full stomach. For example, fat cells produce large amounts of inflammation-causing substances, such as interleukin-6 and C-reactive protein. With two-thirds of the population now overweight, it is easy to see how large numbers of people have set the stage for chronic inflammatory diseases.

Physicians and biomedical researchers are starting to appreciate the significance of the Inflammation Syndrome—how many different inflammatory diseases are interrelated. As one example, being overweight significantly increases the risk of developing diabetes, a disease with a strong undercurrent of inflammation. Both overweight and diabetes increase the risk of coronary artery disease, now recognized as being inflammatory in origin.

What many health professionals have missed, however, is that early signs of inflammation—whether a minor condition, such as gingivitis, or an asymptomatic elevated C-reactive protein level—stimulate inflammation throughout the body, increasing wear and tear and boosting the risk of far more serious inflammatory disorders. Recognizing the early signs of inflammation can be as valuable to us as canaries in cages were to miners a century ago. The canaries provided an early warning of poisonous gas, allowing miners to escape to the surface with their lives. Similarly, paying attention to—and taking action to reverse—minor types inflammation can help us reduce the risk of very serious diseases such as arthritis, heart disease, Alzheimer's disease, and some types of cancer.

Throughout this book, a key message has been stated and restated: our physical bodies, and our health, are directly related to the quality and diversity of nutrients we consume. The situation is analogous to the construction of a house. When quality building materials are used, the house has a sound foundation and structure. When shoddy building materials are used, the foundation and structure are weak and won't last as long.

We can control the quality of nutrients we consume—the building materials of our bodies. We can consume foods that stimulate inflammation, which is unfortunately what the majority of people seem to be doing, or we can eat foods that naturally reduce inflammation.

The Inflammation Syndrome is about making choices that can improve our health. As individuals, we hold our futures in the palms of our hands. We can choose to ignore the evidence and take our chances with long-term health. Or we can take many steps to improve our chances of having a long and healthy life.

Medical Tests to Assess Inflammation

If you would like more precise, medically supervised testing for inflammatory disorders, it might be worthwhile to consult a nutritionally oriented physician. (See appendix B for referral services.) Such a physician is often willing to do a number of tests beyond those of many conventional physicians. Although health maintenance organizations (HMOs) are not likely to cover such services, standard insurance policies may cover part of the costs.

Among the tests that would be helpful are:

- high- or ultrasensitive C-reactive protein to measure systemic inflammation and cardiovascular risk;
- oxidative-stress panel to measure levels of antioxidant vitamins and free radicals;
- fatty acid profile to determine levels of pro- and anti-inflammatory fats;
- food allergy profile, including IgE and IgG reactions, to indicate allergies;
- fecal microbiology test to evaluate pathogens and beneficial bacteria in the gastrointestinal tract;
- intestinal permeability to determine whether leaky gut is contributing to allergylike sensitivities;
- fasting and two-hour glucose and insulin levels to determine whether impaired glucose tolerance and hyperinsulinemia (diabetic and prediabetic condition) are factors in inflammation.

APPENDIX B

Sources of Anti-Inflammatory Products

Nutritional Supplements

Many companies market a variety of anti-inflammatory supplements. Although these companies are not allowed to make a therapeutic claim for nutritional supplements, many of their product names are often very suggestive, and clerks in health food stores and pharmacies can often provide guidance.

Some products are formulated as general anti-inflammatory supplements with many ingredients, whereas others are stand-alone products such as omega-3 fish oil, gamma-linolenic acid (GLA), glucosamine, and vitamin E supplements. The following companies produce and market high-quality products.

ABKIT, Inc.

Abkit manufactures the CamoCare line of skin-care products with chamomile and AlphaBetic, a once-a-day supplement for people with diabetes. Many of these products are available at health food stores, natural foods groceries, and pharmacies. For more information call 800-226-6227 or go to www.abkit.com.

Advanced Physicians Products

Founded by a nutritionally oriented physician, APP offers a broad line of excellent vitamin and mineral supplements, including omega-3 fish oils, natural vitamin E, and many other products. APP also is a source for Coromega fish oils. (See ERBL below.) For more information call 800-220-7687 or go to www.nutritiononline.com.

Bioforce

Bioforce is a Swiss maker of herbal products—mostly tinctures, but also some tablets and ointments. The products are not standardized in the conventional sense, but the company's manufacturing controls ensure consistency and high-quality products. For more information call 877-232-6060 or go to www.bioforce.com.

J. R. Carlson Laboratories

Carlson Laboratories offers the widest selection of natural vitamin E products, including supplements, creams, ointments, suppositories, and more. The company also sells a wide range of other vitamin and mineral supplements, including omega-3 fish oils, GLA, and glucosamine. For more information call toll-free 888-234-5656 or go to www.carlson labs.com.

ERBL

Erbl, Inc., markets Coromega, an orange-flavored omega-3 fish oil supplement that comes in squeezable foil packets, a taste and form factor that often appeals to children. For more information call 877-275-3725 or go to www.coromega.com.

Nature's Way

Nature's Way is a leading herb supplement company, with most of its 350 products sold in capsule form. Some of the company's products are standardized; others are whole herb products. For more information call 801-489-1500 or go to www.naturesway.com.

Nordic Naturals

Nordic Naturals markets a line of high-quality varied fish oil capsules, with slight differences in formulation designed to support joints, the cardiovascular system, and brain function. Some of the products are flavored to mask the "fishy" quality of omega-3 fatty acids. For more information call 800-662-2544 or go to www.nordicnaturals.com.

Nutricology/Allergy Research Group

Nutricology/Allergy Research Group is often at the cutting edge of original and useful nutritional supplements. Its main anti-inflammatory products are Enzocaine and Inflamed. Like most of the other companies listed in this section, it is known for exceptional quality. For more information call 800-545-9960 or go to www.nutricology.com.

Nutrition 21

This company supplies "raw materials" for more familiar brands of supplements. Nutrition 21 is the maker of Chromax chromium picolinate, the form of chromium best documented in clinical trials with diabetic subjects. The company also manufactures Diachrome, a proprietary combination of chromium picolinate and biotin (a B vitamin), which also helps control blood sugar levels. You may find the name Chromax in fine print on the back of supplements. The Nutrition 21 brand of Diachrome can be purchased by calling 800-343-3082 or 914-701-4500, ext. 517.

PharmaNord

This Scandinavian company markets Bio-Sport, which contains anti-inflammatory fish oils and antioxidants. The product has been used extensively in Europe, particularly by the Danish Olympic team to ease inflammatory injuries. It is currently available through limited distribution in the United States. For more information go to www.pharma nord.com.

Pure Scientific

This company markets an expanding line of Advantig brand supplements that preventively target different aspects of inflammation, such as joint, heart, and gastrointestinal health. These are innovative products that address some of the major focal points of inflammatory disorders. For example, the Advantig product for joint health includes many anti-inflammatory nutrients and herbs, including MSM, curcumin, ginseng, quercetin, N-acetylcysteine, green tea, grape seed extract, bromelain, alpha-lipoic acid, carotenoids, and flavonoids. For more information go to www.advantig.net (note the .net address, not .com) or call toll-free 877-877-4566.

Thorne Research

Thorne is one of the most morally ethical supplement companies, and product quality is exceptionally high. The company sells primarily to physicians, but it also accepts orders from consumers (mail order only). Thorne has a broad line of products, including many anti-inflammatory nutrients. Its MediClear product provides nutritional support for inflammation, allergies, and gastrointestinal integrity. For more information call 208-263-1337 or go to www.thorne.com.

UltraBalance Medical Foods

UltraInflamX, which is distributed by Metagenics, Inc., *only to physicians,* is a meal supplement designed with many anti-inflammatory nutrients. Ask your physician to obtain information directly from the company at 800-843-9660 or go to www.ultrabalance.com.

Vitamin Shoppe

This mail order company sells most (not all) leading health food brands of supplements discounted by 25 to 30 percent, which can lead to substantial savings. For more information call 800-223-1216.

Natural Grocers

The Anti-Inflammation Syndrome Diet Plan recommends eating fresh and natural foods. Your best bet for finding meat from range-fed animals and organic fruits and vegetables is a natural foods grocery store such as Wild Oats, Whole Foods, or one of the many independent stores. One of the best independent chains (but without fresh meat or fish) is Vitamin Cottage, with about a dozen stores in Denver and Colorado Springs. Trader Joe's grocery stores also have many high-quality meats, fish, fruits, and vegetables, though they are not always organically produced.

Trader Joe's

Trader Joe's is a chain of offbeat but high-quality "specialty retail" grocery stores, with many organic, gluten-free, and wholesome products.

You won't find the selection of a large supermarket, but the meats, vegetables, and seafood (frozen) are of exceptional quality and at comparatively reasonable prices. For more information and the locations of Trader Joe's stores go to www.traderjoes.com.

Wild Oats

This national chain emphasizes natural and gourmet foods. Wild Oats' meat departments offer free-range meats. For more information call 800-494-WILD or go to www.wildoats.com.

Whole Foods

Like Wild Oats, the emphasis is on wholesome, natural foods, including free-range meats, organic produce, and a wide variety of other healthful food products. For more information go to www.wholefoods.com.

Specialty Foods

Australian Mac Nut Oil

Macadamia nut oil is rich in oleic acid, a beneficial anti-inflammatory omega-9 fat. This product, sold under Dr. Pescatore's Healthy! for Good label, is cold-processed without chemicals. It has a high smoke point, so it can be used (if necessary) at very high stir-frying temperatures. Because of its subtle, nutty aroma, it can be used as an alternative to olive oil. For more information call toll-free 888-350-8446.

Czimer's Game and Seafood

If you live in the Chicago area, you are lucky to be near one of the most venerable purveyors of game meat. Czimer's has been in the retail business for more than thirty-five years, selling venison, bear, antelope, and other game meats. It's open Monday through Saturdays and is at 13136 West 159th Street, Lockport, IL 60441. For more information call 708-301-0500.

Earth Song Whole Foods

Earth Song makes several whole grain (some gluten-free) snack bars that redefine the meaning of a wholesome sweet. Among the bars are apple-walnut and cranberry-orange. In addition, Earth Song blends an excellent gluten-free muesli, known as Grandpa's Secret Omega-3 Muesli, which makes for a tasty and quick breakfast (if you take about five minutes to prepare it the night before). For more information call 877-327-8476 or go to www.earthsongwholefoods.com.

Eggland's Best

Eggland's Best is one of several egg producers that feed their chickens extra vitamins and fatty acids and, as a consequence, get eggs with higher levels of vitamin E and omega-3 fatty acids and lower levels of saturated fats. For more information call 610-265-6500 or go to www.eggland.com.

Greatbeef.com

Greatbeef.com is supported by more than a dozen independent family farmers who humanely raise livestock and chicken. Most of the animals are free-range or pasture-fed, with the result being meat with a natural balance of fatty acids and less saturated fat. Members of Greatbeef.com are in Arizona, California, Colorado, Iowa, Minnesota, Missouri, Nebraska, Nevada, Oregon, Pennsylvania, Tennessee, Texas, and Virginia. For more information about specific ranchers and how to buy meat from them go to www.greatbeef.com.

Lotus Foods

Lotus Foods offers a variety of original and tasty rice and rice flour products, including Bhutanese Red Rice and purple Forbidden Rice. The different rices will enhance your appreciation of rice, and the flours can be used to "bread" fish and chicken as well as to make gluten-free crepes. This company's products are truly exceptional. If your health food store does not carry Lotus Foods' rice and rice flours, ask it to order these products. For more information call 510-525-3137 or go to www. lotusfoods.com to order or to find recipes.

Northwest Natural

Northwest Natural makes frozen salmon burgers, halibut burgers, and tuna with pesto medallions, which can be pan fried or microwaved for a quick lunch (with a side vegetable dish). The company's products are sold by Wild Oats and other natural foods grocers. For more information call 360-866-9661.

Omega Nutrition

Omega Nutrition produces a broad selection of unrefined, organic, and minimally processed cooking oils, which can be shipped directly to your home. For information call 800-661-3529 or go to www.omega flo.com.

Pilgrim's Pride EggsPlus

Pilgrim's Pride, one of the largest egg producers in the United States, offers eggs fortified with omega-3 fatty acids. For more information call 800-824-1159.

Van's International Foods

Van's makes several excellent (and some wheat-free) waffles that can be part of a breakfast or dessert. For example, at breakfast, butter a Van's apple-cinnamon waffle with almond butter. For more information go to www.vansintl.com.

Wild Salmon Sources

Wild salmon contains a higher portion of anti-inflammatory omega-3 fatty acids compared with farmed salmon. By 2004, labeling laws will require distributors to identify the country of origin and whether the salmon was wild or farmed. For now, all types of Alaskan salmon—including king, coho, and sockeye—are always wild. You can also order wild salmon online from takusmokeries.com, alaskafoods.com, copperriver seafood.com, and ilovesalmon.com.

Nutritionally Oriented Organizations and Physicians

American College for Advancement in Medicine

www.acam.org

International Association for Orthomolecular Medicine

www.orthomed.org

American Association of Naturopathic Physicians

www.aanp.org

Health Practitioners Mentioned in This Book

Burton M. Berkson, M.D., Ph.D., Las Cruces, NM; phone: 505-524-3720

Ashton Embry; e-mail: AEmbry@NRCan.gc.ca; Web site: www.direct-ms.org

Abram Hoffer, M.D., Ph.D., Victoria, BC, Canada; phone: 250-386-8756

Ronald E. Hunninghake, M.D., Wichita, KS; phone: 316-682-3100

Judy A. Hutt, N.D., Tucson, AZ; phone: 520-887-4287

Robert S. Ivker, D.O., Denver, CO; phone: 888-434-0033; Web site: www.thrivinghealth.com

Richard Kunin, M.D., San Francisco, CA; phone: 415-346-2500

Shari Lieberman, Ph.D., New York, NY; phone: 212-439-8728

Søren Mavrogenis, Copenhagen, Denmark; phone: 45-33-33-8009; e-mail: cph@centrumfys.dk

Hugh D. Riordan, M.D., Wichita, KS; phone: 316-682-3100

Hunter Yost, M.D., Tucson, AZ; phone: 520-219-5060; Web site: doctor.medscape.com/HunterYostMD

Laboratories for Testing Nutrient Levels

The most scientific way of supplementing is to start by having your levels of vitamins, minerals, and fats measured. In that way you know exactly which nutrients you should increase. Most testing laboratories prefer to work with physicians. These three laboratories are well respected for their analytical capabilities. Physicians can prepare blood for shipment to them.

Bright Spot for Health

316-682-3100

www.brightspot.org

Great Smokies Diagnostic Laboratory

800-522-4762

www.greatsmokies-lab.com

Pantox Laboratories

619-272-3885

www.pantox.com

Newsletters, Magazines, Books, and Web Sites

Many publications provide excellent information on diet and supplements, though sometimes you may have to navigate contradictory information or ignore information inconsistent with the Anti-Inflammation Syndrome Diet Plan.

Newsletters and Magazines

The Nutrition Reporter

This monthly newsletter, produced by Jack Challem (the author of this book), summarizes recent research on vitamins, minerals, and herbs. The annual subscription rate is $26 ($48 CND for Canada, $38 U.S. funds for all other countries). For a sample issue, send a business-size self-addressed envelope, with postage for two ounces, to *The Nutrition Reporter,* P.O. Box 30246, Tucson, AZ 85751. Sample issues also are available at www.nutritionreporter.com.

Let's Live

This monthly magazine focuses on how diet, nutrition, and supplements help maintain health and reverse disease. The annual subscription is $15.95. To order, call 800-365-3790.

Natural Health

Natural Health eclectically covers the entire range of natural health—supplements, herbs, home remedies, diet, food, and lifestyle. Its articles are well researched and thorough. The annual subscription is $17.95. To order, call 800-526-8440.

Books

Syndrome X: The Complete Nutritional Program to Prevent and Reverse Insulin Resistance by Jack Challem, Burton Berkson, M.D., Ph.D., and Melissa Diane Smith (New York: John Wiley & Sons, 2000; $14.95). With a diet program similar to the Anti-Inflammation Syndrome Diet Plan, *Syndrome X* focuses more on preventing diabetes and heart disease, as well as losing weight.

The Paleo Diet by Loren Cordain, Ph.D. (New York: John Wiley & Sons, 2001; $24.95). Cordain, one of the leading experts on the Paleolithic diet, describes that diet, which can be considered the original Anti-Inflammation Syndrome Diet Plan.

Why Grassfed Is Best!: The Surprising Benefits of Grassfed Meat, Eggs, and Dairy Products by Jo Robinson (Vashon, WA: Vashon Island Press, 2000; $7.50). This small book (128 pages) is worth every penny. It makes a powerful case for eating grassfed meats and other foods, most of which are compatible with the Anti-Inflammation Syndrome Diet Plan. Included is a list of sources for meat from free-range and pasture-fed animals. Order it from Vashon Island Press, 29428 129th Avenue SW, Vashon, WA 98070. For more information call 206-463-4156. You also can order it from www.thestoreforhealthyliving.com. Add $4.50 for shipping and handling.

Going Against the Grain: How Reducing and Avoiding Grains Can Revitalize Your Health by Melissa Diane Smith (Chicago: Contemporary Books, 2002; $14.95). This book explores how the cultivation and consumption of grains led to a deterioration in people's health. Smith provides dietary plans for having low-grain and zero-grain diets.

Know Your Fats: The Complete Primer for Understanding the Nutrition of Fats, Oils, and Cholesterol by Mary G. Enig, Ph.D. (Silver Spring, MD: Bethesda Press, 2000; $29.95). Though technical, *Know Your Fats* may be the most comprehensive consumer book on making sense of the many dietary fats. For more information e-mail customer@bethesda press.com or go to bethesdapress.com.

Web Sites

The Official Anti-Inflammation Syndrome Diet Plan Web Site
www.stopinflammation.com

The Nutrition Reporter
Dozens of articles on vitamins and minerals.
www.nutritionreporter.com

Consumerlab.com
Independent reports evaluating whether specific nutritional supplements contain what their labels say. Although Consumerlab.com performs fair and independent evaluations, it tests only a small percentage of the nutritional supplements on the market, and it identifies only those that pass (not those that fail) testing.
www.consumerlab.com

Medline
The world's largest database of medical journal articles, providing free abstracts (summaries) of more than 8 million articles.
www.ncbi.nlm.nih.gov

Melissa Diane Smith
Nutrition consultant and expert on the health hazards of grains, including information from the book *Going Against the Grain*.
www.melissadianesmith.com

Merck Manual
The online edition of your physician's standard medical reference book.
www.merck.com

Nutrient Data Laboratory Food Composition
Type in nearly any food or food product and you instantly get its nutritional breakdown per cup or 100 grams.
www.nal.usda.gov/fnic/foodcomp/

Paleo Diet/Recipes
Most of these modern verions of Paleolithic recipes are compatible with the Anti-Inflammation Syndrome Diet Plan.
www.panix.com/~paleodiet/list/

Price-Pottenger Foundation
A Web site dedicated to two twentieth-century nutritional pioneers.
www.price-pottenger.org

SELECTED REFERENCES

1. Meet the Inflammation Syndrome

Lindmark, E., et al. "Relationship between Interleukin-6 and Mortality in Patients with Unstable Coronary Artery Disease: Effects of an Early Invasive or Noninvasive Strategy." *JAMA* 288 (2001): 2107–2113.

Page J, and D. Henry, "Consumption of NSAIDs and the Development of Congestive Heart Failure in Elderly Patients: An Underrecognized Public Health Problem." *Archives of Internal Medicine* 160 (2000): 777–784.

Shield, M. "Anti-Inflammatory Drugs and Their Effects on Cartilage Synthesis and Renal Function." *European Journal of Rheumatology & Inflammation* 13 (1993): 7–16.

Zhang, R., et al. "Association between Myeloperoxidase Levels and Risk of Coronary Artery Disease." *JAMA* 286 (2001): 2136–2142.

2. Your Inflammation Triggers

Espinola-Klein, C., et al. "Impact of Infectious Burden on Extent and Long-Term Prognosis of Atherosclerosis." *Circulation* 105 (2002): 15–21.

Hadjivassiliou, M., et al. "Headache and CNS White Matter Abnormalities Associated with Gluten Sensitivity." *Neurology* 56 (2001): 385–388.

Kirjavainen, P., and G. R. Gibson. "Healthy Gut Microflora and Allergy: Factors Influencing Development of the Microbiotica." *Annals of Medicine* 31 (1999): 288–292.

Léone, J., et al. "Rheumatic Manifestations of Scurvy: A Report of Two Cases." *Revue du Rhumatisme* (English ed.) 64 (1997): 428–431.

Purba, M., et al. "Skin wrinkling: Can Food Make a Difference?" *Journal of the American College of Nutrition* 20 (2001): 71–80.

3. The Dietary Causes of Inflammation

Choy, E. H. S., and G. S. Panayi. "Cytokine Pathways and Joint Inflammation in Rheumatoid Arthritis." *New England Journal of Medicine* 344 (2001): 907–916.

Cohen, H. A., I. Neuman, and H. Nahaum. "Blocking Effect of Vitamin C in Exercise-Induced Asthma." *Archives of Pediatric and Adolescent Medicine,* 151 (1997): 467–470.

Darlington, L. G., and T. W. Stone. "Antioxidants and Fatty Acids in the Amelioration of Rheumatoid Arthritis and Related Disorders." *British Journal of Nutrition* 85 (2001): 251–269.

Enig, M. G. *Know Your Fats: The Complete Primer for Understanding the Nutrition of Fats, Oils, and Cholesterol.* Silver Spring, MD: Bethesda Press, 2000.

Grimble, R. F. "Modification of Inflammatory Aspects of Immune Function by Nutrients." *Nutrition Research* 18 (1998): 1297–1317.

———. "Nutritional Modulation of Cytokine Biology." *Nutrition* 14 (1998): 634–640.

Heller, A., et al. "Lipid Mediators in Inflammatory Disorders." *Drugs* 55 (1998): 487–496.

Hu, F. B., et al. "Dietary Fat Intake and Risk of Coronary Heart Disease in Women." *New England Journal of Medicine* 337 (1997): 1491–1499.

Hwang, D. "Essential Fatty Acids and Immune Response." *FASEB Journal* 3 (1989): 2052–2061.

Kankaanpaa, Sutas Y., et al. "Dietary Fatty Acids and Allergy." *Annals of Medicine* 31 (1999): 282–287.

Neuman, I., H. Nahum, and A. Ben-Amotz. "Prevention of Exercise-Induced Asthma by a Natural Isomer Mixture of B-Carotene." *Annals of Allergy, Asthma, and Immunology* 82 (1999): 549–553.

———. "Reduction of Exercise-Induced Asthma Oxidative Stress by Lycopene, A Natural Antioxidant." *Allergy* 55 (2000): 1184–1189.

Toborek, M., et al. "Unsaturated Fatty Acids Selectively Induce an Inflammatory Environment in Human Endothelial Cells." *American Journal of Clinical Nutrition* 75 (2002): 119–125.

Wu, D., M. G. Hayek, and S. N. Meydani. "Vitamin E and Macrophage Cyclooxygenase Regulation in the Aged." *Journal of Nutrition* 131 (2001): 382S–388S.

4. Balancing a Diet That's Out of Balance

Cordain, L., et al. "Plant-Animal Subsistence Ratios and Macronutrient Energy Estimates in Worldwide Hunter-Gatherer Diets." *American Journal of Clinical Nutrition* 71 (2000): 682–692.

de Vegt, F., et al. "Relation of Impaired Fasting and Postload Glucose with Incident Type 2 Diabetes in a Dutch Population." *JAMA* 285 (2001): 2109–2113.

Gerster, H. "Can Adults Adequately Convert A-linolenic Acid (18:3n-3) to Eicosapentaenoic Acid (20:5n-3) and Docosahenxaenoic Acid (22:6n-3)?" *International Journal of Vitamin and Mineral Research* 68 (1998): 159–173.

Hall, R. S. *Food for Nought: The Decline in Nutrition.* New York: Harper & Row, 1974.

Howell, W. H. "Diet and Blood Lipids." *Nutrition Today* 32 (1997): 110–115.

Khaw, K. T., et al. "Glycated Haemoglobin, Diabetes, and Mortality in Men in Norfolk Cohort of European Prospective Investigation of Cancer and Nutrition (EPIC-Norfolk)." *BMJ* 322 (2001): 15–18.

Subar, A. F., et al. "Dietary Sources of Nutrients among U.S. Adults, 1989 to 1991." *Journal of the American Dietetic Association* 98 (1998): 537–547.

5. What's Wrong with Anti-Inflammatory Drugs

Angell, M. "Is Academic Medicine for Sale?" *New England Journal of Medicine* 342 (2000): 1516–1518.

Chew, L. D., et al. "A Physician's Survey of the Effect of Drug Sample Availability on Physician's Behavior." *Journal of General Internal Medicine* 15 (2000): 478–483.

Bliznakov, E. G., and D. J. Wilkins. "Biochemical and Clinical Consequences of Inhibiting Coenzyme Q_{10} Biosynthesis by Lipid-Lowering HMG-CoA Reductase Inhibitors (Statins): A Critical Overview." *Advances in Therapy* 15 (1998): 218–228.

Bodenheimer, T. "Uneasy Alliance: Clinical Investigators and the Pharmaceutical Industry." *New England Journal of Medicine* 342 (2000): 1539–1544.

Bombardier, P., et al. "Comparison of Upper Gastrointestinal Toxicity of Rofecoxib and Naproxen in Patients with Rheumatoid Arthritis." *New England Journal of Medicine* 343 (2000): 1520–1528.

Brandt, K. D. "Should Nonsteroidal Anti-Inflammatory Drugs Be Used to Treat Osteoarthritis?" *Rheumatic Diseases Clinics of North America* 19 (1993): 29–44.

Gamlin, L., and J. Brostoff. "Food Sensitivity and Rheumatoid Arthritis." *Environmental Toxicology and Pharmacology* 4 (1997): 43–49.

Hoffer, L. J., et al. "Sulfate Could Mediate the Therapeutic Effect of Glucosamine Sulfate." *Metabolism* 50 (2001): 767–770.

Hollon, M. F. "Direct-to-Consumer Marketing of Prescription Drugs: Creating Consumer Demand." *JAMA* 281 (1999): 382–384.

Horton, R. "Lotronex and the FDA: A Fatal Erosion of Integrity." *Lancet* 357 (2001): 1544–1545.

Lazarou, J., B. H. Pomeranz, and P. N. Corey. "Incidence of Adverse Drug Reactions in Hospitalized Patients." *JAMA* 279 (1998): 1200–1205.

Lichtenstein, D. R., and M. M. Wolfe. "Cox-2-selective NSAIDs: New and Improved?" *JAMA* 284 (2000): 1297–1299.

Lockwood, K., et al. "Progress on Therapy of Breast Cancer with Vitamin Q_{10} and the Regression of Metastases." *Biochemical and Biophysical Research Communications* 212 (1995): 172–177.

Mendelsohn, R. S. *Confessions of a Medical Heretic.* Chicago: Contemporary Books, 1979.

Mukherjee, D., S. E. Nissen, and E. J. Topol. "Risk of Cardiovascular Events Associated with Selective Cox-2-Inhibitors." *JAMA* 286 (2001): 954–959.

Overvad, K., et al. "Coenzyme Q_{10} in Health and Disease." *European Journal of Clinical Nutrition* 53 (1999): 764–770.

Page, J., and D. Henry. "Consumption of NSAIDs and the Development of Congestive Heart Failure in Elderly Patients: An Underrecognized Public Health Problem." *Archives of Internal Medicine* 160 (2000): 777–784.

Phillips, D. P., N. Christenfeld, and L. M. Glynn. "Increase in U.S. Medication-Error Deaths between 1983 and 1993." *Lancet* 351 (1998): 643–644.

Portakal, O., et al. "Coenzyme Q_{10} Concentrations and Antioxidant Status in Tissues of Breast Cancer Patients." *Clinical Biochemistry* 33 (2000): 279–284.

Rao, C. V., H. L. Newmark, and B. S. Reddy. "Chemopreventive Effect of Squalene on Colon Cancer." *Carcinogenesis* 19 (1998): 287–290.

Relman, A. S. "Separating Continuing Medical Education from Pharmaceutical Marketing." *JAMA* 285 (2001): 1009–1012.

Ridker, P. M., et al. "C-reactive Protein and Other Markers of Inflammation in the Prediction of Cardiovascular Disease in Women." *New England Journal of Medicine* 342 (2000): 836–843.

Shield, M. J. "Anti-Inflammatory Drugs and Their Effects on Cartilage Synthesis and Renal Function." *European Journal of Rheumatology & Inflammation,* 13 (1993): 7–16.

Shorr, R. I., and W. L. Greene. "A Foodborne Outbreak of Expensive Antibiotic Use in a Community Teaching Hospital." *Journal of the American Medical Association* 273 (1995): 1908.

Simon, L. S., et al. "Anti-Inflammatory and Upper Gastrointestinal Effects of Celecoxib in Rheumatoid Arthritis: A Randomized Controlled Trial." *JAMA* 282 (1999): 1921–1928.

Stolberg, S. G. "Now, Prescribing Just What the Patient Ordered." *New York Times,* August 10, 1997, E3.

Vane, J. R., Y. S. Bakhle, and R. M. Botting. "Cyclooxygenases 1 and 2." *Annual Review of Pharmacology and Toxicology* 38 (1998): 97–120.

Washington, S. O. "Drug Company Lies about Celebrex in *JAMA.*" *Washington Post,* August 5, 2001, A11.

Wolfe, M. M., D. R. Lichtenstein, and G. Singh. "Gastrointestinal Toxicity of Nonsteroidal Anti-Inflammatory Drugs." *New England Journal of Medicine* 340 (1999): 1888–1899.

Woodman, R. "*Lancet:* FDA Far Too Cozy with Drug Industry." Reuters News Service, May 18, 2001.

6. Fifteen Steps to Fight the Inflammation Syndrome

Blacklock, C. J., et al. "Salicylic Acid in the Serum of Subjects Not Taking Aspirin: Comparison of Salicylic Acid Concentrations in the Serum of Vegetarians, Nonvegetarians, and Patients Taking Low-Dose Aspirin." *Journal of Clinical Pathology* 54 (2001): 553–555.

Eberhardt, M. V., C. Y. Lee, and R. H. Liu. "Antioxidant Activity of Fresh Apples." *Nature* 405 (2000): 903–904.

Guillemant, J., et al. "Mineral Water as a Source of Dietary Calcium: Acute Effects on Parathyroid Function and Bone Resorption in Young Men." *American Journal of Clinical Nutrition* 71 (2000): 999–1002.

Liu, S. et al. "A High-Glycemic Diet in Relation to Plasma Levels of High-Sensitivity C-Reactive Protein in Middle-Aged Women." *American Journal of Epidemiology* 153, supp. 11 (2001): S97.

Pauling, L. "Orthomolecular Psychiatry." *Science* 160 (1968): 265–271.

Szent-Gyorgyi, A. V. *On Oxidation, Fermentation, Vitamins, Health, and Disease.* Baltimore: Williams & Wilkins, 1939.

Travis, J. "Mice Reveal the Off Switch for Inflammation." *Science News* 160 (2001): 388.

Yudkin, J. S., et al. "C-Reactive Protein in Healthy Subjects: Associations with Obesity, Insulin Resistance, and Endothelial Dysfunction: A Potential Role for Cytokines Originating from Adipose Tissue?" *Arteriosclerosis, Thrombosis, and Vascular Biology* 19 (1999): 72–78.

8. Good Fats That Rev Up Your Body's Natural Anti-Inflammatories

Bagga, D., et al. "Dietary Modulation of Omega-3/Omega-6 Polyunsaturated Fatty Acid Ratios in Patients with Breast Cancer." *Journal of the National Cancer Institute* 89 (1997): 1123–1131.

Bell, R. R., M. J. Spencer, and J. L. Sherriff. "Voluntary Exercise and Monounsaturated Canola Oil Reduce Fat gain in Mice Fed Diets High in Fat." *Journal of Nutrition* 127 (1997): 2006–2010.

Belluzzi, A., et al. "Effect of an Enteric-Coated Fish-Oil Preparation on Relapses in Crohn's Disease." *New England Journal of Medicine* 334 (1996): 1557–1560.

Conner, W. E. "N-3 Fatty Acids from Fish and Fish Oil: Panacea or Nostrum?" *American Journal of Clinical Nutrition* 74 (2001): 415–416.

Curtis, C. L., et al. "N-3 Fatty Acids Specifically Modulate Catabolic Factors Involved in Articular Cartilage Degradation." *Journal of Biological Chemistry* 275 (2000): 721–724.

Dewailly, E., et al. "N-3 Fatty Acids and Cardiovascular Disease Risk Factors among the Inuit of Nunavik." *American Journal of Clinical Nutrition* 74 (2001): 464–473.

Ernst, E., T. Saradeth, and G. Achhammer. "N-3 Fatty Acids and Acute-Phase Proteins." *European Journal of Clinical Investigation* 21 (1991): 77–82.

Faarvang, K. L., et al. "Fish Oils and Rheumatoid Arthritis: A Randomized and Double-Blind Study." *Ugeskrift for Lager* 156 (1994): 3495–3498.

Ferrara, L. A., et al. "Olive Oil and Reduced Need for Antihypertensive Medications." *Archives of Internal Medicine* 160 (2000): 837–842.

Hubbard, N. E., D. Lim, and K. L. Erickson. "Alteration of Murine Mammary

Tumorigenesis by Dietary Enrichment with n-3 Fatty Acids in Fish Oil." *Cancer Letters* 124 (1998): 1–7.

Iso, H., et al. "Intake of Fish and Omega-3 Fatty Acids and Risk of Stroke in Women." *JAMA* 285 (2001): 304–312.

James, M. J., R. A. Gibson, and L. G. Cleland. "Dietary Polyunsaturated Fatty Acids and Inflammatory Mediator Production." *American Journal of Clinical Nutrition* 71 (Suppl.) (2000): 343S–348S.

Jolly, C. A., et al. "Life Span Is Prolonged in Food-Restricted Autoimmune-Prone (NZB x NZW) F(1) Mice Fed a Diet Enriched with (n-3) Fatty Acids." *Journal of Nutrition* 131 (2001): 2753–2760.

Kunin, R. A. "Snake Oil: A Potent Source of Omega-3 EFA." *Journal of Orthomolecular Medicine* 4 (1989): 139–140.

Lau, C. S., K. D. Morley, and J. J. F. Belch. "Effects of Fish Oil Supplementation on Nonsteroidal Anti-Inflammatory Drug Requirement in Patients with Mild Rheumatoid Arthritis: A Double-Blind Placebo-Controlled Study." *British Journal of Rheumatology* 32 (1993): 982–989.

Leventhal, L. L., E. G. Boyce, and R. B. Zurier. "Treatment of Rheumatoid Arthritis with Gammalinolenic Acid." *Annals of Internal Medicine* 9 (1993): 867–873.

Linos, A., et al. "Dietary Factors in Relation to Rheumatoid Arthritis: A Role for Olive Oil and Cooked Vegetables." *American Journal of Clinical Nutrition* 70 (1999): 1077–1082.

Lorgeril, M. de, et al. "Mediterranean Diet, Traditional Risk Factors, and the Rate of Cardiovascular Complications after Myocardial Infarction." *Circulation* 99 (1999): 779–785.

Mantzioris, E., et al. "Biochemical Effects of a Diet Containing Foods Enriched with n-3 Fatty Acids." *American Journal of Clinical Nutrition* 72 (2000): 42–48.

Prakash, C., et al. "Decreased Systematic Thromboxane A2 Biosynthesis in Normal Human Subjects Fed a Salmon-Rich Diet." *American Journal of Clinical Nutrition* 60 (1994): 369–373.

Requirand, P., et al. "Serum Fatty Acid Imblanace in Bone Loss: Example of Periodontal Disease." *Clinical Nutrition* 19 (2000): 271–276.

Rose, D. P. "Dietary Fatty Acids and Cancer." *American Journal of Clinical Nutrition* 66 (1997): 998S–1003S.

Shapiro, J. A., et al. "Diet and Rheumatoid Arthritis in Women: A Possible Protective Effect of Fish Consumption." *Epidemiology* 7 (1996): 256–263.

Stoll, A. L., W. E. Severus, and M. P. Freeman. "Omega-3 Fatty Acids in Bipolar Disorder: A Preliminary Double-Blind, Placebo-Controlled Trial." *Archives of General Psychiatry* 56 (1999): 407–412.

Terry, P., et al. "Fatty Fish Consumption and Risk of Prostate Cancer." *Lancet* 357 (2001): 1764–1766.

Visioli, F., and C. Galli. "The Effect of Minor Constituents of Olive Oil on Cardiovascular Disease: New Findings." *Nutrition Reviews* 56 (1998): 142–147.

Wolk, A., et al. "A Prospective Study of Association of Monounsaturated Fat and Other Types of Fat with Risk of Breast Cancer." *Archives of Internal Medicine* 158 (1998): 41–45.

Wu, D., et al. "Effect of Dietary Supplementation with Black Currant Seed Oil on the Immune Response of Healthy Elderly Subjects." *American Journal of Clinical Nutrition* 70 (1999): 536–543.

Yaqoob, P., et al. "Effect of Olive Oil on Immune Function in Middle-Aged Men." *American Journal of Clinical Nutrition* 67 (1998): 129–135.

Zurier, R. B., et al. "Gamma-Linolenic Acid Treatment of Rheumatoid Arthritis: A Randomized, Placebo-Controlled Study." *Arthritis & Rheumatism* 11 (1996): 1808–1817.

9. Vitamin E to Extinguish the Flames of Inflammation

Chan, A. C. "Vitamin E and Atherosclerosis." *Journal of Nutrition* 128 (1998): 1593–1596.

Darlington, L. G., and T. W. Stone. "Antioxidants and Fatty Acids in the Amelioration of Rheumatoid Arthritis and Related Disorders." *British Journal of Nutrition* 85 (2000): 251–269.

Devarai, S., and I. Jialal. "Alpha-Tocopherol Decreases Interleukin-1b Release from Activated Human Monocytes by Inhibition of 5-Lipoxygenase." *Arteriosclerosis Thrombosis and Vascular Biology* 19 (1999): 1125–1133.

———. "Alpha-tocopherol Supplementation Decreases Serum C-Reactive Protein and Monocyte Interleukin-6 Levels in Normal Volunteers and Type 2 Diabetic Patients." *Free Radical Biology & Medicine* 29 (2000): 790–792.

———. "Low-Density Lipoprotein Postsecretory Modification, Monocyte Function, and Circulating Adhesion Molecules in Type 2 Diabetes Patients with and without Macovascular Complications: The Effect of A-Tocopherol Supplementation." *Circulation* 102 (2000): 191–196.

Edmonds, S. E., et al. "Putative Analgesic Activity of Repeated Oral Doses of Vitamin E in the Treatment of Rheumatoid Arthritis: Results of a Prospective Placebo-Controlled Double-Blind Trial." *Annals of the Rheumatic Diseases* 56 (1997): 649–655.

Fogarty, A., et al. "Dietary Vitamin E, IgE Concentrations, and Atopy." *Lancet* 356 (2000): 1573–1574.

Helmy, M., et al. "Antioxidants as Adjuvant Therapy in Rheumatoid Disease: A Preliminary Study." *Arzneimittel-Forschung/Drug Research* 51 (2001): 293–298.

Islam, K. N., S. Devaraj, and I. Jialal. "Alpha-Tocopherol Enrichment of Monocytes Decreases Agonist-Induced Adhesion to Human Endothelial Cells." *Circulation* 98 (1998): 2255–2261.

Jialal, I., M. Traber, and S. Deveraj. "Is There a Vitamin E Paradox?" *Current Opinion in Lipidology* 12 (2001): 49–53.

Jiang, Q., and B. N. Ames. "In Vivo Anti-Inflammatory Effect of Gamma-Tocopherol." *Free Radical Biology & Medicine* 31 (Suppl.) (Abstract 123) (2001): 47.

Kennedy, M., et al. "Successful and Sustained Treatment of Chronic Radiation Proctitis with Antioxidant Vitamins E and C." *American Journal of Gastroenterology* 96 (2001): 1080–1084.

Meydani, S. N., et al. "Vitamin E Supplementation and in Vivo Immune Response in Healthy Elderly Subjects." *JAMA* 277 (1997): 1380–1386.

Sano, M., et al. "A Controlled Trial of Selegiline, Alpha-Tocopherol, or Both as Treatment for Alzheimer's Disease." *New England Journal of Medicine* 336 (1997): 1216–1222.

Stephens, N. G., et al. "Randomized Controlled Trial of Vitamin E in Patients with Coronary Disease: Cambridge Heart Antioxidant Study (CHAOS)." *Lancet* 347 (1996): 781–786.

Uomo, G., G. Talamini, and P. G. Rabitti. "Antioxidant Treatment in Hereditary Pancreatitis: A Pilot Study on Three Young Patients." *Digestive and Liver Diseases* 33 (2001): 58–62.

Upritchard, J. E., W. H. F. Sutherland, and J. I. Mann. "Effect of Supplementation with Tomato Juice, Vitamin E, and Vitamin C on LDL Oxidation and Products of Inflammatory Activity in Type 2 Diabetes." *Diabetes Care* 23 (2000): 733–738.

Valigra, L. "Vitamin E May Stop Alzheimer's Cell Death." UPI newswire, August 27, 1999.

van Tits, L. J., et al. "Alpha-Tocopherol Supplementatin Decreases Production of Superoxide and Cytokines by Leukocytes ex Vivo in Both Normolipidemic and Hypertriglyceridemic Individuals." *American Journal of Clinical Nutrition* 71 (2000): 458–464.

Zheng, K. C., et al. "Effect of Dietary Vitamin E Supplementation on Murine Nasal Allergy." *American Journal of the Medical Sciencies* 318 (1999): 49–54.

10. Glucosamine, Chondroitin, and Vitamin C to Rebuild Your Tissues

Adams, M. E. "Hype about Glucosamine." *Lancet* 354 (1999): 353–354.

Challem, J. J. "Did the Loss of Endogenous Ascorbate Propel the Evolution of Anthropoidea and *Homo sapiens?*" *Medical Hypotheses* 48 (1997): 387–392.

Challem, J. J., and E. W. Taylor. "Retroviruses, Ascorbate, and Mutations in the Evolution of *Homo sapiens.*" *Free Radical Biology & Medicine* 25 (1995): 130–132.

Cumming, A. "Glucosamine in Osteoarthritis." *Lancet* 354 (1999): 1640–1641.

Das, A Jr., and T. A. Hammad. "Efficacy of a Combination of FCHG49 Glucosamine Hydrochloride, TRH122 Low Molecular Weight Sodium Chondroitin Sulfate, and Manganese Ascorbate in the Management of Knee Osteoarthritis." *Osteoarthritis and Cartilage* 8 (2000): 343–350.

Hoffer, L. J., et al. "Sulfate Could Mediate the Therapeutic Effect of Glucosamine Sulfate." *Metabolism,* 50 (2001): 767–770.

Johnston, C. S., and L. L. Thompson. "Vitamin C Status of an Outpatient Population." *Journal of the American College of Nutrition* 17 (1998): 366–370.

Langlois, M., et al. "Serum Vitamin C Concentration Is Low in Peripheral Arterial Disease and Is Associated with Inflammation and Severity of Artherosclerosis." *Circulation* 103 (2001): 1863–1868.

Leffler, C. T., et al. "Glucosamine, Chondroitin, and Manganese Ascorbate for Degenerative Joint Disease of the Knee or Low Back: A Randomized, Double-Blind, Placebo-Controlled Pilot Study." *Military Medicine* 164 (1999): 85–91.

Leone, J., et al. "Rheumatic Manifestations of Scurvy: A Report of Two Cases." *Revue du Rhumatisme* (English ed.) 64 (1997): 428–431.

Reginster, J. Y., et al. "Long-Term Effects of Glucosamine Sulphate on Osteoarthritis Progression: A Randomised Placebo-Controlled Clinical Trial." *Lancet* 357 (2001): 247–248, 251–256.

Ronca, F., et al. "Anti-inflammatory Activity of Chondroitin Sulfate." *Osteoarthritis and Cartilage* 6 (Suppl. A) (1998): 14–21.

Rovati, L. C., M. Annefeld, and G. Giacovelli. "Glucosamine in Osteoarthritis." *Lancet* 354 (1999): 1640.

Russell, A. I., and M. F. McCarty. "Glucosamine in Osteoarthritis." *Lancet* 354 (1999): 1641.

Shankland, W. E. II. "The Effects of Glucosamine and Chondroitin Sulfate on Osteoarthritis of the TMJ: A Preliminary Report of 50 Patients." *Orofacial Pain* 16 (1999): 230–235.

11. B Vitamins and More to Reduce Inflammation

Bayeta, E., and B. H. S. Lau. "Pycnogenol Inhibits Generation of Inflammatory Mediators in Macrophages." *Nutrition Research* 20 (2000): 249–259.

Berkson, B. M. "A Conservative Triple Antioxidant Approach to the Treatment of Hepatitis C." *Medizinische Klinik* 94 (Suppl. 3) (1999): 84–89.

Bernard, M. A., P. A. Nakonezny, and T. M. Kashner. "The Effect of Vitamin B_{12} on Older Veterans and Its Relationship in Health." *Journal of the American Geriatrics Society* 46 (1998): 1199–1206.

Blacklock, C. J., et al. "Salicylic Acid in the Serum of Subjects Not Taking Aspirin: Comparison of Salicylic Acid Concentrations in the Serum of Vegetarians, Nonvegetarians, and Patients Taking Low-Dose Aspirin." *Journal of Clinical Pathology* 54 (2000): 553–555.

Chantre, P., et al. "Efficacy and Tolerance of *Haroagophytum procumbens* versus Diacerhein in Treatment of Osteoarthritis." *Phytomedicine* 7 (2000): 177–183.

Cho, K. J., et al. "Inhibition Mechanisms of Bioflavonoids Extracted from the Bark of *Pinus maritima* on the Expression of Pro-inflammatory Cytokines." *Healthy Aging for Functional Longevity* 928 (2001): 141–156.

De Flora, S., C. Grassi, and L. Carati. "Attenuation of Influenza like Symptomatology and Improvement of Cell-Mediated Immunity with Long-Term

N-acetylcysteine Treatment." *European Respiratory Journal* 10 (1997): 1535–1541.

Eberhardt, M. V., C. Y. Lee, and R. H. Liu. "Antioxidant Activity of Fresh Apples." *Nature* 405 (2000): 903–904.

Erlinger, T. P., et al. "Relationship between Systemic Markers of Inflammation and Serum Beta-Carotene Levels." *Archives of Internal Medicine* 161 (2000): 1903–1908.

Haqqi, T. M., et al. "Prevention of Collagen-Induced Arthritis in Mice by a Polyphenolic Fraction from Green Tea." *Proceedings of the National Academy of Sciences* 96 (1999): 4524–4529.

Jurna, I. "Analgesic and Analgesia-Potentiating Action of B Vitamins." *Schermz* 12 (1998): 136–141.

Kritchevsky, S. B., et al. "Serum Carotenoids and Markers of Inflammation in Nonsmokers." *American Journal of Epidemiology* 152 (2000): 1065–1071.

Kwok, B. H., et al. "The Anti-Inflammatory Natural Product Parthenolide from the Medicinal Herb Feverfew Directly Binds to and Inhibits IkappaB kinase." *Chemistry and Biology* (2001): 759–766.

Li, W. G., et al. "Anti-Inflammatory Effect and Mechanism of Proanthocyanidins from Grape Seeds." *Acta Pharmacologica Sinica* 22 (2001): 1117–1120.

Middleton, E., and Anne S. "Quercetin Inhibits Lipopolysaccharide-Induced Expression of Endothelial Cell Tracellular Adhesion Molecule-1." *International Archives of Allergy and Immunology* 107 (1995): 435–436.

Panasenko, O. M. et al. "Interaction of Peroxynitrite with Carotenoids in Human Low-Density Lipoproteins." *Archives of Biochemistry and Biophysics* 373 (2000): 302–305.

Ringbom, Segura L., et al. "Usolic Acid from Plantago Major, a Selective Inhibitor of Cyclooxygenase-2 Catalyzed Prostaglandin Biosynthesis." *Journal of Natural Products* 61 (1998): 1212–1215.

Sandoval-Chacon, M., et al. "Antiinflammatory Actions of Cat's Claw: The Role of NF-kB." *Alimentary Pharmacology and Therapeutics* 12 (1998): 1279–1289.

Srivastava K. C., and T. Mustafa. "Ginger *(Zingiber offinale)* in Rheumatism and Musculoskeletal Disorders." *Medical Hypotheses* 39 (1992): 342–348.

Stefanescu, M., et al. "Pycnogenol Efficacy in the Treatment of Systemic Lupus Erythematosus Patients." *Phytotherapy Research* 15 (2001): 698–704.

Wegener, T. "Devil's claw: From African Traditional Remedy to Modern Analgesic and Anti-Inflammatory." *HerbalGram* 50 (2001): 1047–1054.

Weisburger, J. H. "Tea and Health: A Historical Perspective." *Cancer Letters* 114 (1997): 315–317.

Zakay-Rones, Z., et al. "Inhibition of Several Strains of Influenza Virus in Vitro and Reduction of Symptoms by an Elderberry Extract *(Sambucus nigra L.)* during an Outbreak of Influenza B Panama." *Journal of Alternative and Complementary Medicine* 1 (1995): 361–369.

12. The Inflammation Syndrome, Diseases, and Specific Conditions

Altman, R. D., and K. C. Marcussen. "Effects of a Ginger Extract on Knee Pain in Patients with Osteoarthritis." *Arthritis & Rheumatism* 44 (2001): 2531–2538.

Anderson, R. A., et al. "Elevated Intakes of Supplemental Chromium Improve Glucose and Insulin Variables in Individuals with Type 2 Diabetes." *Diabetes* 46 (1997): 1786–1791.

Angswurm, M. W., et al. "Selenium Replacement in Patients with Severe Systemic Inflammatory Response Syndrome Improves Clinical Outcome." *Critical Care Medicine* 27 (1999): 1807–1813.

Anon. "The Scourge of Boomeritis." *My Generation* (September/October 2001): 14.

Beck, M. A., et al. "Rapid Genomic Evolution of a Nonvirulent Coxsackievirus B$_3$ in Selenium-Deficient Mice Results in Selection of Identical Virulent Isolates." *Nature Medicine* 1 (May 1995): 433–436.

Bell, R. R., M. J. Spencer, and J. L. Sherriff. "Voluntary Exercise and Monounsaturated Canola Oil Reduce Fat Gain in Mice Fed Diets High in Fat." *Journal of Nutrition* 127 (1997): 2006–2010.

Berkson, B. M. "A Conservative Triple Antioxidant Approach to the Treatment of Hepatitis C." *Medizinische Klinik* 94 (Supp. III) (1999): 84–89.

Brinkeborn, R., et al. "Echinaforce in the Treatment of Acute Colds." *Schweizerische Zeitschrift für Ganzheits Medizin* 10 (1998): 26–29.

Burger, R. A., A. R. Torres, and R. P. Warren. "Echinacea-Induced Cytokine Production by Human Macrophages." *International Journal of Immunopharmacology* 19 (1997): 371–379.

Chan, A. C. "Vitamin E and Atherosclerosis." *Journal of Nutrition* 128 (1998): 1593–1596.

Cheraskin, E. "How Quickly Does Diet Make for Change? A Study in Gingival Inflammation." *New York Journal of Denistry* 58 (1998): 133–135.

Chongviriyaphan, N., X. D. Wang, and R. M. Russell. "The Effects of a Combination of Antioxidant Vitamins on Lung Squamous Metaplasia and Lipid Peroxidation in Ferrets Exposed to Tobacco Smoke." Presented at the 42nd annual meeting of the American College of Nutrition, October 4–7, Orlando, Florida.

Clark, L. C., et al. "Effects of Selenium Supplementation for Cancer Prevention in Patients with Carcinoma of the Skin: A Randomized Controlled Trial." Nutritional Prevention of Cancer Study Group. *JAMA* 276 (1996): 1957–1963.

Cohen, H. A., I. Neuman, and H. Nahaum. "Blocking Effect of Vitamin C in Exercise-Induced Asthma." *Archives of Pediatric and Adolescent Medicine* 151 (1997): 467–470.

Cohen, M. E., and D. M. Meyer. "Effect of Dietary Vitamin E Supplementation and Rotational Stress on Alveolar Bone Loss in Rice Rats." *Archives of Oral Biology* 38 (1993): 601–606.

Cook, D. G., et al. "Effect of Fresh Fruit Consumption on Lung Function and Wheeze in Children." *Thorax* 52 (1997): 628–633.

Cordain, L., et al. "Modulation of Immune Function by Dietary Lectins in Rheumatoid Arthritis." *British Journal of Nutrition* 83 (2000): 207–217.

Correa, P., et al. "Chemoprevention of Gastric Dysplasia: Randomized Trial of Antioxidant Supplements and Anti-Helicobacter Pylori Therapy." *Journal of the National Cancer Institute* 92 (2000): 1881–1888.

Cowley, H. C., et al. "Plasma Antioxidant Potential in Severe Sepsis: A Comparison of Survivors and Nonsurvivors." *Critical Care Medicine* 24 (1996): 1179–1183.

Curtis, C. L., et al. "N-3 Fatty Acids Specifically Modulate Catabolic Factors Involved in Articular Cartilage Degradation." *Journal of Biological Chemistry* 275 (2000): 721–724.

De Flora, S., C. Grassi, and L. Carati. "Attenuation of Influenzalike Symptomatology and Improvement of Cell-Mediated Immunity with Long-Term N-Acetylcysteine Treatment." *European Respiratory Journal* 10 (1997): 1535–1541.

Eberlein-Konig, B., M. Placzek, and B. Przybilla. "Protective Effect against Sunburn of Combined Systemic Ascorbic Acid (Vitamin C) And D-a-tocopherol (Vitamin E)." *Journal of the American Academy of Dermatology* 38 (1998): 45–48.

Festa, A., et al. "Chronic Subclinical Inflammation as Part of the Insulin Resistance Syndrome: The Insulin Resistance Atherosclerosis Study (IRAS)." *Circulation* 102 (2000): 42–47.

Field, A. E., et al. "Impact of Overweight on the Risk of Developing Common Chronic Diseases during a Ten-Year Period." *Archives of Internal Medicine* 161 (2001): 1581–1586.

Flynn, M. A., W. Iirvin, and G. Krause. "The Effect of Folate and Cobalamin on Osteoarthritic Hands." *Journal of the American College of Nutrition* 13 (1994): 351–356.

Fraser, A. G., and G. A. Woollard. "Gastric Juice Ascorbic Acid Is Related to *Helicobacter pylori* Infection but Not Ethnicity." *Journal of Gastroenterology and Hepatology* 14 (1999): 1070–1073.

Gadek, J. E., S. J. DeMichele, and M. D. Karlstad. "Effect of Enteral Feeding with Eicoapentaenoic Acid, Gamma-Linolenic Acid, and Antioxidants in Patients with Acute Respiratory Distress Syndrome." *Critical Care Medicine* 27 (1999): 1409–1420.

Gamlin, L., and J. Brostoff. "Food Sensitivity and Rheumatoid Arthritis." *Environmental Toxicology and Pharmacology* 4 (1997): 43–49.

Giovannucci, E. "Tomatoes, Tomato-Based Products, Lycopene, and Cancer: Review of the Epidemiology Literature." *Journal of the National Cancer Institute* 91 (1999): 317–331.

Giovannucci, E., et al. "Intake of Carotenoids and Retinol in Relation to Risk of Prostate Cancer." *Journal of the National Cancer Institute* 87 (1995): 1767–1776.

Golding, D. N. "Is There an Allergic Synovitis?" *Journal of the Royal Society of Medicine* 83 (1990): 312–314.

Gollnick, H. P. M., et al. "Systemic Beta-Carotene plus Topical UV-Sunscreen Are an Optimal Protection against Harmful Effects of Natural UV-Sunlight: Results of the Berlin-Eilath Study." *European Journal of Dermatology* 6 (1996): 200–205.

Gonzalez N. J., and L. L. Isaacs. "Evaluation of Pancreatic Proteolytic Enzyme Treatment of Adenocarcinoma of the Pancreas, with Nutrition and Detoxification Support." *Nutrition and Cancer* 33 (1999): 117–124.

Guochang, A. "Ultraviolet Radiation-Induced Oxidative Stress in Cultured Human Skin Fibroblasts and Antioxidant Protection." *Biological Research Reports from the University of Jyväskylä* 33 (1993): 1–86.

Hadjivassiliou, M., et al. "Headache and CNS White Matter Abnormalities Associated with Gluten Sensitivity." *Neurology* 56 (2001): 385–388.

Hafstrom, I., et al. "A Vegan Diet Free of Gluten Improves the Signs and Symptoms of Rheumatoid Arthritis: The Effects on Arthritis Correlate with a Reduction in Antibodies to Food Antigens." *Rheumatology* 40 (2001): 1175–1179.

Haney, D. O. "Tomato Nutrient May Fight Cancer." Associated Press, April 13, 1999.

Hanioka, T., et al. "Effect of Topical Application of Coenzyme Q_{10} on Adult Periodontitis." *Molecular Aspects of Medicine* 15 (1994): S241–S248.

Haqqi, T. M., et al. "Prevention of Colagen-Induced Arthritis in Mice by a Polyphenolic Fraction from Green Tea." *Proceedings of the National Academy of Sciences* 96 (1999): 4524–4529.

Hayes, C. E., M. T. Cantorna, and H. F. DeLuca. "Vitamin D and Multiple Sclerosis." *Proceedings of the Society for Experimental Biology & Medicine* 216 (1997): 21–27.

Hemila, H. "Does Vitamin C Alleviate the Symptoms of the Common Cold? A Review of Current Evidence." *Scandinavian Journal of Infectious Diseases* 26 (January 1994): 1–6.

Herzenberg, L. A., et al. "Glutathione Deficiency Is Associated with Impaired Survival in HIV Disease." *Proceedings of the National Academy of Sciences of the USA* 94 (1997): 1967–1972.

Hodge, L., J. K. Peat, and C. Salome. "Increased Consumption of Polyunsaturated Oils May Be a Cause of Increased Prevalence of Children Asthma." *Australia and New Zealand Journal of Medicine* 24 (1994): 727.

Hodge, L., et al. "Consumption of Oily Fish and Childhood Asthma Risk." *Medical Journal of Australia* 164 (1996): 137–140.

Hoffer, A., and L. Pauling. "Hardin Jones Biostatistical Analysis of Mortality Data for a Second Set of Cohorts of Cancer Patients with a Large Fraction Surviving at the Termination of the Study and a Comparison of Survival Times of Cancer Patients Receiving Large Regular Oral Doses of Vitamin

C and Other Nutrients with Similar Patients Not Receiving These Doses." *Journal of Orthomolecular Medicine* 8 (1993): 157–167.

Hogan, S. P., et al. "A Pathological Function for Eotaxin and Eosinophils in Eosinophilic Gastrointestinal Inflammation." *Nature Immunology* 2 (2001): 353–360.

Hosseini, S., et al. "Pycnogenol in the Management of Asthma." *Journal of Medicinal Food* 4 (2001): 201–209.

Hutter, C. "On the Causes of Multiple Sclerosis." *Medical Hypotheses* 41 (1993): 93–96.

Huisman, A. M., et al. "Vitamin D Levels in Women with Systemic Lupus Erythematosus and Fibromyalgia." *Journal of Rheumatology* 28 (2001): 2535–2539.

Jacob, R. A., et al. "Experimental Vitamin C Depletion and Supplementation in Young Men: Nutrient Interactions and Dental Health Effects." *Annals of the New York Academy of Sciences* 498 (1987): 333–346.

Jarosz, M., et al. "Effects of High-Dose Vitamin C Treatment on *Helicobacter pylori* Infection and Total Vitamin C Concentration in Gastric Juice." *European Journal of Cancer Prevention* 7 (1998): 449–454.

Kira, J., S. Tobimatsu, and I. Goto. "Vitamin B_{12} Metabolism and Massive-Dose Methyl Vitamin B_{12} Therapy in Japanese Patients with Multiple Sclerosis." *Internal Medicine* 33 (1994): 82–86.

Kirjavainen, P., and G. R. Gibson. "Healthy Gut Microflora and Allergy: Factors Influencing Development of the Microbiotica." *Annals of Medicine* 31 (1999): 288–292.

Kjeldsen-Kragh, J., et al. "Controlled Trial of Fasting and One-Year Vegetarian Diet in Rheumatoid Arthritis." *Lancet* 338 (1991): 899–902.

Krohn, J. The *Whole Way to Allergy Relief & Prevention*. Point Roberts, Wash.: Hartley & Marks, 1991.

Lamm, D. L., et al. "Megaose Vitamins in Bladder Cancer: A Double-Blind Clinical Trial." *The Journal of Urology* 151 (1994): 21–26.

Lau, C. S., K. D. Morley, and J. J. F. Belch. "Effects of Fish Oil Supplementation on Nonsteroidal Anti-Inflammatory Drug Requirement in Patients with Mild Rheumatoid Arthritis: A Double-Blind Placebo-Controlled Study." *British Journal of Rheumatology* 32 (1993): 982–989.

MacNee, W., and I. Rahman. "Oxidants and Antioxidants as Therapeutic Targets in Chronic Obstructive Pulmonary Disease." *American Journal of Critical Care Medicine* 160 (1999): S58–S65.

Madsen, T., et al. "C-Reactive Protein, Dietary n-3 Fatty Acids, and the Extent of Coronary Artery Disease." *American Journal of Cardiology* 88 (2001): 1139–1142.

Maire, F., et al. "Factors Associated with Hyperhomocysteinemia in Crohn's Disease." *Gastroenterologie Clinique et Biologique* 25 (2001): 745–748.

McVean, M., and D. C. Liebler. "Inhibition of UVB-Induced DNA Photodamage in Mouse Epidermis by Topically Applied A-tocopherol." *Carcinogenesis* 18 (1997): 1617–1622.

Messetti, A., et al. "Systemic Oxidative Stress and Its Relationship with Age and Illness." *Journal of the American Geriatrics Society* 44 (1996): 823–827.

Milam, S. B., G. Zardeneta, and J. P. Schmitz. "Oxidative Stress and Degenerative Temporomandibular Joint Disease: A Proposed Hypothesis." *Journal of Oral and Maxillofacial Therapy* 56 (1998): 214–223.

Miller, A. L. "The Etiologies, Pathophysiology, and Alternative/Complementary Treatment of Asthma." *Alternative Medicine Review* 6 (2001): 20–47.

Nair, S., et al. "Micronutrient Antioxidants in Gastric Mucosa and Serum in Patients with Gastritis and Gastric Ulcer." *Journal of Clinical Gastroenterology* 30 (2000): 381–385.

Nelson, H. K., et al. "Host Nutritional Selenium Status as a Driving Force for Influenza Virus Mutations." *FASEB Journal* 15 (2001): 1481–1483.

Neuman, I., H. Nahum, and A. Ben-Amotz. "Prevention of Exercise-Induced Asthma by a Natural Isomer Mixture of B-Carotene." *Annals of Allergy, Asthma, and Immunology* 82 (1999): 549–553.

———. "Reduction of Exercise-Induced Asthma Oxidative Stress by Lycopene, a Natural Antioxidant." *Allergy* 55 (2000): 1184–1189.

Nordvik, I., et al. "Effect of Dietary Advice and n-3 Supplementation in Newly Diagnosed MS Patients." *Acta Neurologica Scandinavica* 102 (2000): 143–149.

Nsouli, T. M., et al. "Role of Food Allergy in Serous Otitis Media." *Annals of Allergy* 73 (1994): 215–219.

Patavino, T., and D. M. Brady. "Natural Medicine and Nutritional Therapy as an Alternative Treatment in Systemic Lupus Erythematosus." *Alternative Medicine Review* 6 (2001): 460–471.

Patterson, R. E., et al. "Vitamin Supplements and Cancer Risk: The Epidemiological Evidence." *Cancer Causes and Control* 8 (1997): 786–802.

Purba, M., et al. "Skin Wrinkling: Can Food Make a Difference?" *Journal of the American College of Nutrition* 20 (2001): 71–80.

Romieu, I., F. Meneses, and M. Ramirez. "Antioxidant Supplementation and Respiratory Functions among Workers Exposed to High Levels of Ozone." *American Journal of Critical Care Medicine* 158 (1998): 226–232.

Salam, T. N., and J. F. Fowler Jr. "Balsam-Related Systemic Contact Dermatitis." *Journal of the American Academy of Dermatology* 45 (2001): 377–381.

Sano, M., et al. "A Controlled Trial of Selegiline, Alpha-Tocopherol, or Both as Treatment for Alzheimer's Disease." *New England Journal of Medicine* 336 (1997): 1216–1222.

Schnyder, G., et al. "Decreased Rate of Coronary Restenosis after Lowering of Plasma Homocysteine Levels." *New England Journal of Medicine* 345 (2001): 1593–1600.

Schünemann, H. J., et al. "The Relation of Serum Levels of Antioxidant Vitamins C and E, Retinol and Carotenoids with Pulmonary Function in the General Population." *American Journal of Respiratory and Critical Care Medicine* 163 (2001): 1246–1255.

Shankland, W. E. II. "The Effects of Glucosamine and Chondroitin Sulfate on

Osteoarthritis of the TMJ: "A preliminary Report of Fifty Patients." *Orofacial Pain* 16 (1999): 230–235.

Sivam, G. P., et al. "Protection against *Helicobacter pylori* and Other Bacterial Infections by Garlic." Presented at Recent Advances on the Nutritional Benefits Accompanying the Use of Garlic as a Supplement, November 14–17, 1998, Newport Beach, Calif.

Slattery, M. L., et al. "Trans-Fatty Acids and Colon Cancer." *Nutrition and Cancer: An International Journal,* 39 (2001): 170–175.

Stefanescu, M., et al. "Pycnogenol Efficacy in the Treatment of Systemic Lupus Erythematosus Patients." *Phytotherapy Research* 15 (2001): 698–704.

Symons, M. C. R. "Radicals Generated by Bone Cutting and Fracture." *Free Radical Biology & Medicine* 20 (1996): 831–835.

Tixier, J. M., et al. "Evidence by in Vivo and in Vitro Studies That Binding of Pycnogenol to Elastin Affects Its Rate of Degradation by Elastases." *Biochemical Pharmacology* 33 (1984): 3933–3939.

Trenga, C. A., J. Q. Koenig, and P. V. Williams "Dietary Antioxidants and Ozone-Induced Bronchial Hyperresponsiveness in Adults with Asthma." *Archives of Environmental Health* 56 (2001): 242–249.

Vaananen, M. K., et al. "Periodontal Health Related to Plasma Ascorbic Acid." *Proceedings of the Finnish Dental Society* 89 (1993): 51–59.

Wang, Q., W. Z. Zhao, and C. G. Ma. "Protective Effects of Ginkgo Biloba on Gastric Mucosa." *Acta Pharmacologica Sinica* 21 (2000): 1153–1156.

Welch, H. G., L. M. Schwartz, and S. Woloshin. "Are Increasing Five-Year Survival Rates Evidence of Success against Cancer?" *JAMA* 283 (2000): 2975–2978.

Wendland, B. E., et al. "Lipid Peroxidation and Plasma Antioxidant Micronutrients in Crohn Disease." *American Journal of Clinical Nutrition* 74 (2001): 259–264.

Wilson, A. C., et al. "Relation of Infant Diet to Childhood Health: Seven-Year Follow-up of Cohort of Children in Dundee Infant Feeding Study." *British Medical Journal* 316 (1998): 21–25.

Woodward, N., H. Turnstall-Pedoe, and K. McColl. "*Helicobacter pylori* Infection Reduces Systemic Availability of Dietary Vitamin C." *European Journal of Gastroenterology & Hepatology* 13 (2001): 233–237.

Zuerier, R. B., et al. "Gamma-Linolenic Acid Treatment of Rheumatoid Arthritis: A Randomized, Placebo-Controlled Study." *Arthritis & Rheumatism* 11 (1996): 1808–1817.

Zullo, A., V. Rinaldi, and C. Hassan: "Ascorbic Acid and Intestinal Metaplasia in the Stomach: A Prospective Randomized Study." *Alimentary Pharmacology and Therapeutics* 14 (2000): 1303–1309.

INDEX

ABOUT THE AUTHOR

Jack Challem, The Nutrition Reporter, is one of the leading health reporters in the United States. He has been writing about advances in vitamin and mineral research since 1974 and is the lead author of the best-selling *Syndrome X: The Complete Nutritional Program to Prevent and Reverse Insulin Resistance* (New York: John Wiley & Sons, 2000). Challem writes and publishes *The Nutrition Reporter* newsletter (www.nutritionreporter.com) and is a contributing editor to many health and consumer magazines, including *Natural Health, Let's Live,* and *Modern Maturity.* His scientific articles have appeared in *Cosmetic Dermatology, Free Radical Biology & Medicine, Journal of the National Cancer Institute, Journal of Orthomolecular Medicine, Medical Hypotheses,* and the *New England Journal of Medicine.*